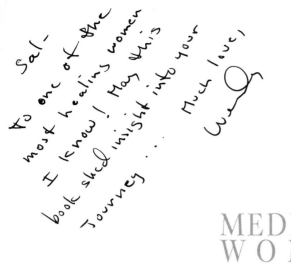

Sal—
To one of the
most healing women
I know! May this
book shed insight into your
journey . . . Much love,

MEDICINE
WOMEN

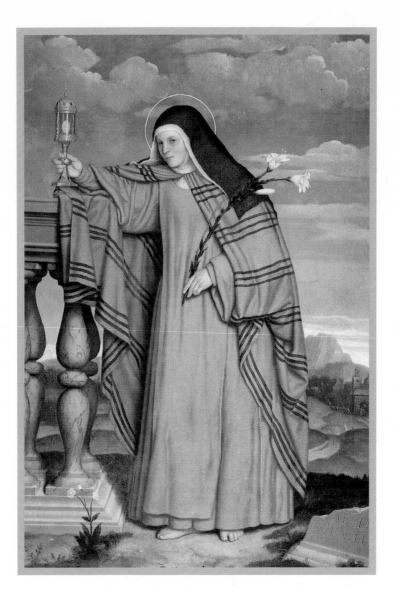

ABOVE: Saint Clare holding a monstrance against the armies of Frederick II by *Giovan Battista Moroni* (1520–78).

MEDICINE WOMEN

A Pictorial History of Women Healers

Elisabeth Brooke

A publication supported by
THE KERN FOUNDATION

Quest Books
Theosophical Publishing House
Wheaton, Illinois ♦ Madras, India

First Quest edition 1997
Co-published with Godsfield Press 1997

For additional information write to:
Quest Books
The Theosophical Publishing House, P.O. Box 270
Wheaton, IL 60189–0270

A publication of the Theosophical Publishing House,
a department of the Theosophical Society in America

This publication was made possible with the assistance
of the Kern Foundation.

DESIGNED AND PRODUCED BY
THE BRIDGEWATER BOOK COMPANY LIMITED

Picture research by Lynda Marshall

Library of Congress Cataloging-in-Publication Data

Brooke, Elisabeth.
    Medicine women: a pictorial history of women healers / Elisabeth
Brooke.
        p.   cm.
    ISBN 0-8356-0751-8
    1. Women in medicine.   2. Women healers.   I. Title.
    R692.B758   1997
    610'. 82--dc20   96-44733
                                                     CIP

Printed and bound in Hong Kong

The publishers wish to thank the following for the use of pictures:
Bridgeman Art Library: pp. 6 Museé Des Beaux-Arts, Rennes; 8 Bibliothèque Nationale, Paris;
11 Whitford and Hughes, London; 12 Louvre, Paris; 19 University of Bologna; 26 San
Francesco Upper Church, Assisi; 31 British Library, London; 38/39 British Library,
London; 41 Louvre, Paris; 44 British Library, London; 70/71 Wallace Collection, London;
80/81 Chiesa Di Santa Maria Novella, Florence; 94 Claydon House, Buckinghamshire; 112
Bibliothèque Nationale, Paris; 117 Private Collection. *e.t.archive:* pp. 2, 20, 47, 62, 78, 101,
108/109. *Hulton-Getty Collection:* pp. 24, 42, 52/53, 68, 79, 83, 103, 114. *Hutchison Library:*
p. 24. *Images:* p. 23. *Marie Stopes International:* pp. 55, 56, 58. *National Library of Jamaica:* p. 104.
National Museums and Art Galleries on Merseyside: pp. 96, 98. *Quest Books, Illinois:* p. 123. *Shocken Books,*
New York/Illustration: Ted Berstein: p. 60. *Wellcome Institute Library, London:* p. 34.
Every effort has been made to contact copyright holders. The publishers would like to
apologize for any inadvertent omissions, and will be pleased to correct these in
subsequent editions.

FRONT COVER: The March Marigold, 1870
by *Sir Edward Burne-Jones* (1833–98),
Piccadilly Gallery/Bridgeman Art Library, London.

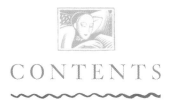

CONTENTS

~~~~~~~~~~

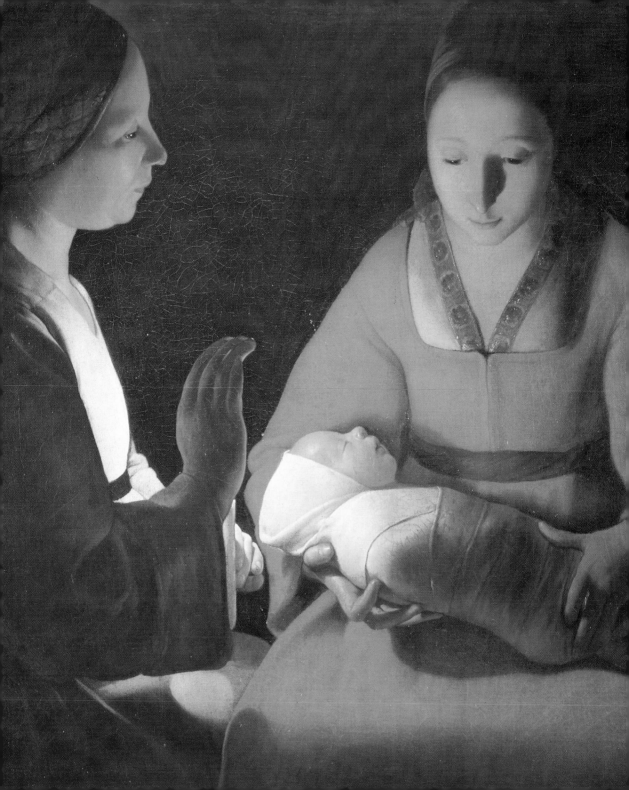

INTRODUCTION

~~~~~~~~~~~~~~~~~~~~

OMEN have always been healers. From the hedge-witch in medieval times and the priestess-healers in Egyptian temples to present-day holistic healers in communities worldwide, they have practiced their healing arts. As the principal provider of care in her family, woman has traditionally had responsibility for the still-room (where medicines were made, plants dried, and alcohol brewed) and the herb garden and has played a vital healing role in the local community. She is the natural midwife and nurse.

What is less well known is that early on women were "professionals" in medicine. They were doctors, professors of medicine, and medical researchers. Women have been at the forefront of medical practice for millennia. It was a woman, Lady Montagu, who introduced smallpox vaccine to Europe, having watched Turkish women inoculating their children. In the nineteenth century the Boston Women's Hospital, run and financed by women, managed to eradicate childbed fever through antiseptic practices long before the medical establishment was prepared to acknowledge the germ theory.

LEFT: The Newborn Child by Georges de La Tour (1593–1652).

It was a woman, Mrs. Hutton, who used purple foxglove to treat water retention due to heart failure, but the man who bought the recipe from her, Dr. Withering, was credited with its discovery.

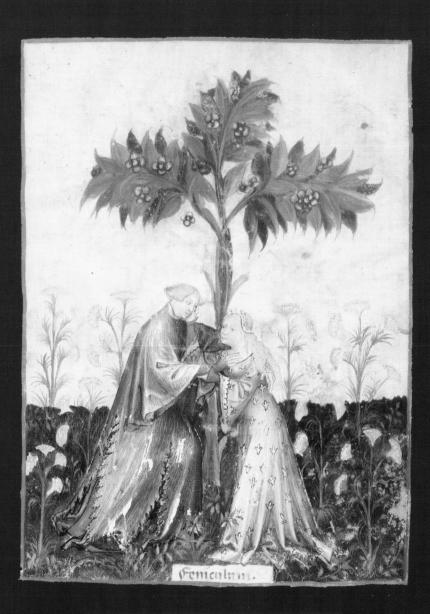

Femenlum.

ABOVE: *Women have traditionally been responsible
for the herb garden. Here fennel is represented in the Tacuinum
Sanitatis of the early fifteenth century.*

Many other medical advances by women have been attributed to men. The most famous case is that of Trotula, a female professor of medicine at Salerno in the eleventh century. A renowned and respected physician, she wrote a detailed book on the diseases of women and children, which was to remain a medical classic for over five hundred years. When our Victorian forefathers were writing up the history of medicine, their misogynous blindness did not permit them to include Trotula as a woman doctor – they claimed it had all been a mistake and that she was a man. Recent scholarly investigation has shown this to be untrue.

Throughout history women have been persecuted for practicing medicine. In fourth-century Athens, Agnodice was sentenced to death for being a doctor, and only the protests of her influential women patients saved her life. In twelfth-century Paris, Jacoba Felice was excommunicated when jealous male colleagues reported her to the bishops, who found her guilty not of malpractice, but simply of being female and a physician – a prohibited combination. Between the fourteenth and the seventeenth centuries there was an orchestrated and thorough campaign to stamp out the woman healer, be she peasant or nobility. The Church, the legal profession, and the newly organized medical profession joined ranks to block her at every turn.

Independent women were recognized as a threat to the power of these organizations, and many thousands – perhaps millions of them – died as a result of the witch-craze. In the nineteenth century there were long and vicious battles to prevent women from entering medical school, with men claiming that women would devalue the profession, but in fact they triumphed in the exams and outshone their churlish male classmates.

A common thread is seen in women's actual practice of medicine. Women are found working in free clinics, running their own hospitals, working in unpopular areas such as public health and geriatrics. They are interested in preventive medicine, in diet – an area long scorned by male doctors – and in the "softer" areas of medicine. Particularly well represented in the area of complementary medicine, women pioneers, such as Mary Baker Eddy and Maria Montessori, stand out. Among traditional healers, women play the vital role that they always have; Mama Lola, for instance, although she lives in New York, carries on the healing traditions within the Voodoo religion that her great-grandmother brought from Africa. The *sangoma* of southern Africa, the *curanderas* of New Mexico, and women shamans continue to practice their native healing rituals.

In its earliest days the Christian Church saw medicine as part of its ministry. Women worked alongside men and opened hospitals for the poor, homes for the aged and maternity units. Throughout the Middle Ages monks and nuns provided medical care for those unable to pay for expensive male doctors. Several Christian women stand out: Hildegard of Bingen, St. Elizabeth of Hungary, Fabiola of Rome. The cult of the Virgin Mary remains to this day a powerful symbol of the healing powers of the feminine, and miracles such as those at Lourdes might be included in the healing work of women.

In the field of midwifery, women have always promoted the gentle, the safe, and the most natural as best for mother and child. Often going against the teachings of the Church, which preached that pain in childbirth was "Eve's curse" and as such should not be alleviated, women have advocated sensible, no-nonsense midwifery. In the seventeenth century an English midwife, Mrs. Cellier, proposed a national network of maternity hospitals, with experienced midwives giving on-the-spot training to students. Her ideas were taken up two hundred years later by Florence Nightingale when she took over the running of a nursing clinic in London. And, writing in the eleventh century, Trotula describes the best way to wean a baby and how important it is not to frighten a woman in labor. Such gentle remedies contrast with the brutal and bloody forceps and stirrup births that became popular from the eighteenth century onwards, and from which midwifery is only just recovering.

In the chapter on remedies I discuss in some detail the healing practices of two women healers. One works with therapeutic touch, a technique that she herself developed and uses in hospitals in the United States, working with qualified nurses. The other example is of a Native American healing ceremony, using peyote and ritual, for Native Americans separated from their tradition. Both of these women healers respect the complex nature of illness and, in their healing work, treat the

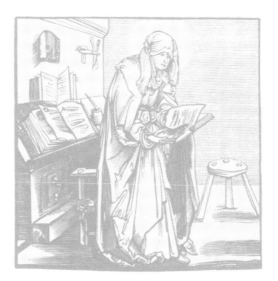

ABOVE: *During the Middle Ages nuns, such as the one in this sixteenth-century wood engraving, played a vital medical role.*

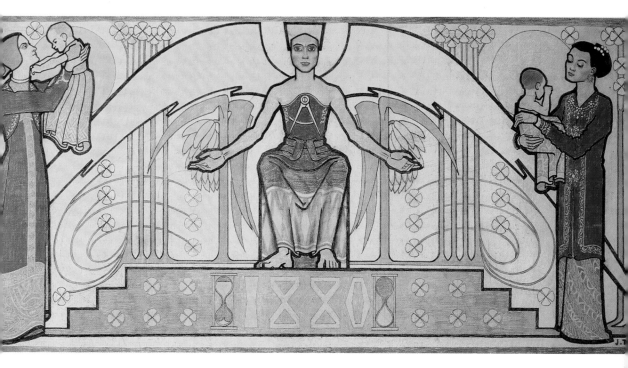

ABOVE: Life's Guardian
by Jan Theodoor Toorop
(1858–1928).

whole person – mind/body/spirit, with emphasis on the spirit.

The Great Goddess, the Healing Mother, Mother Earth, reigned in the hearts and minds of peoples throughout the world many thousands of years before monotheistic religion brought in the concept of God the Father. As Mother Nature, she was the natural protectress of the weak, the sick, and the vulnerable. Throughout history people have invoked the Great Mother in healing rituals and have used her power to heal disease. In the late twentieth century we have come full circle and are now looking to reintegrate the spiritual into our healing traditions, remembering our healing past.

NB DATING: BCE: BEFORE THE COMMON ERA, I.E., BC **CE:** COMMON ERA, I.E., AD

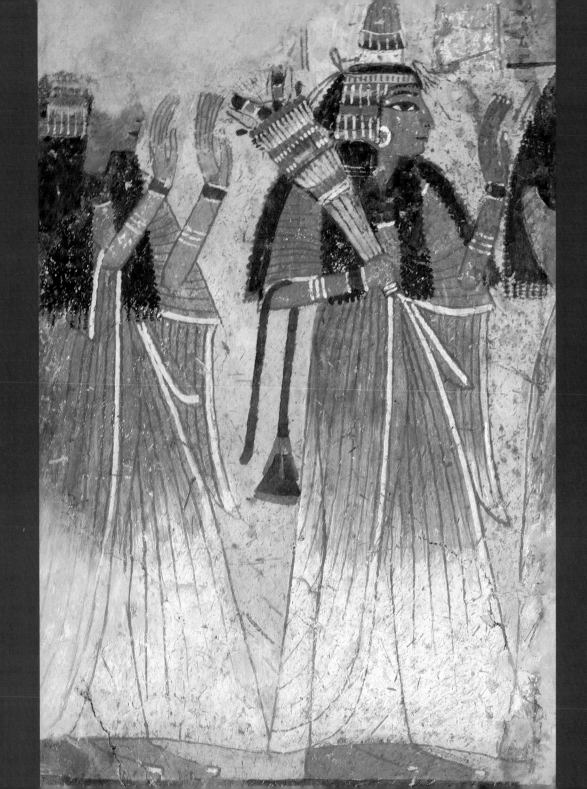

THE GODDESS
AS HEALER

REDATING Christianity by thousands of years, Goddess worship revered and valued the feminine principle. Indeed, Robert Briffault, writing on the Goddess, considers early culture to be very much the product of the feminine.[1] Many early activities, such as food preparation, weaving, pottery, and medicine, were handed down secretly from mother to daughter, and those engaging in these skills had to undergo special preparation. Ritual and prayers were developed to accompany the various stages and activities of life.

As the primary providers of care, women reared children, nursed the sick, and took care of the dying. Woman was seen as the source of life, mother and guardian of the tribe. Her body swelled in pregnancy, she bled each month but did not die from her "wound," and she produced milk that nourished the helpless infant. All these functions were seen as mysteries, connected in some way with the waxing and waning of the moon: women in close-knit groups tend to menstruate in tandem, a pregnancy lasts nine moon cycles, and women's moods change with the moon. So the moon, women, and the sacred became associated.

Without children the tribe could not continue, so naturally the pregnant woman became sacred. Throughout the world statues have been found depicting pregnant women, which were probably

LEFT: *Women, here shown in procession in an Egyptian wall painting, held high status in Egypt.*

---

1. *THE MOTHERS*, VOL. 1, ROBERT BRIFFAULT, LONDON AND NEW YORK, 1927, PP.447–90.

worshiped as part of a fertility cult. Woman was seen as the embodiment of power and was associated with the abundance of the Earth and with life itself.

As the provider of care, woman naturally needed to find remedies for illnesses. She no doubt experimented with the roots, leaves, and berries she came across as her tribe moved about. And when fire was discovered, these simple remedies would have been cooked or mixed together. This was a kind of magic, and as goddess of the food-giving plants, herbs, and fruits, woman numinously transformed these basic elements. She was thus the inventor and guardian of the first healing potions, medicines, and poisons.[2]

As societies became settled, her rudimentary skills would have been refined. Some women would have been seen as especially skilled in healing and would have been consulted by others and perhaps revered for their special powers or their knowledge. But always the Goddess or life energy would have been viewed behind the miracles. Life being unpredictable, and human beings small and vulnerable in the face of nature, the protection and approval of the Mother Goddess would have been sought at especially dangerous times: pregnancy, childbirth, infancy, sickness, and so on. Prayers would have been sent up, sacrifices made, sacred, beautiful objects gathered in her

name, altars and shrines constructed. Women would have been the natural guardians of such places, and they would have worked to interpret the omens and advise on the offerings. Thus a goddess-centered society was born, and the servers or priestesses also became the healers, the midwives, and the layers out of the dead.

It was not until the establishment of the monotheistic religions – Judaism, Christianity, Islam – whose principal God was heavenly and male, that women began to be forbidden public office and prevented from working in the professions.

THE HEALING TEMPLES OF EGYPT

Around 4000 BCE a dynasty of queens was established in Egypt. The Egyptians had two classes of gods – those who were purely spiritual and, best beloved, those who had been human but, through some special act, were admitted to the assembly of gods.

Isis was of the second category; the daughter of Geb and Nut, she was believed to have been a woman who, in an earlier time, had rendered an invaluable service to the Egyptian people. She was their earliest lawmaker and, through her teaching, the Egyptians rose from barbarism to civilization.

---

2. *THE GREAT MOTHER*, ERICH NEUMANN, BOLLINGER, PRINCETON, 1972, P.286.

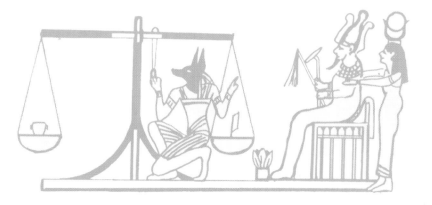

LEFT: Isis, the Divine Mother, here standing behind the throne of Osiris, was a skilled physician.

The science of medicine was said to have originated with Isis. Her name meant Light, Life, and statues of Isis bore this description: "I am all that has been, and all that shall be, and none among mortals has hitherto taken off my veil."[3]

Isis worship was universal among Egyptians, and her temples were magnificent. Her priestesses, consecrated to purity, had to bathe daily, wore linen robes free from animal fiber, and were strict vegetarians. The most sacred mysteries of the Egyptian religion, whose secrets even Pythagoras could not penetrate, were known only to the highest order of priestesses, those of Isis. Moses, "learned in the wisdom of the Egyptians," borrowed much from Isis.

Women held high status in Egypt, and priestesses were recruited from the ranks of the nobility. Ramses III had this inscription engraved on his monuments: "To unprotected woman there is freedom to wander through the whole country wheresoever she list without apprehending danger."[4]

Egypt was the cradle of the medical temple, although it is not known when these began. Isis, the Divine Mother, was especially skilled in the diseases of women and children, and her priestesses were also physicians. They used "rational" medicine, herbs, massages, baths, and so on, and combined them with the "irrational medicine" of prayer, incantations, and ritual. Many temple complexes were huge and resembled health spas, with people traveling long distances to be treated. The largest was the Temple of Isis at Kopto; those at Saïs and Heliopolis also flourished, and later on important medical schools were established.

The *Papyrus Ebers* (named after its finder) was dedicated to Isis: "As it is to be, a thousand times.

3. *WOMAN, CHURCH AND STATE*, MATILDA GAGE, 1893, REPRINTED BY PERSEPHONE PRESS, WATERTOWN, MASS., 1980, P.16. 4. GAGE, NEW EDITION, P.18.

This is the book for the healing of all diseases. May Isis heal me as she healed Horus."[5] It is dated around 1550 BCE and contains hundreds of prescriptions, many of them for women's diseases. The *Kahun Papyrus*, dated around 1900 BCE, also covers the diseases of women and children. Since only women practitioners treated female diseases, this was clearly a text for women doctors, probably those from Saïs. Records have been found of a woman doctor practicing in the reign of Neferirika-ra, around 2730 BCE, who was believed to have been working at Saïs.

GODDESS HEALING IN A PRE-CHRISTIAN SOCIETY

It is believed that the Sumerians, living on the banks of the Tigris and the Euphrates, were the first to evolve a theory of demons causing disease. Their culture existed 6,000 years ago and was highly developed. In the grave of Queen Shubad of Ur, 3500 BCE, were found prescriptions for stopping pain written on clay tablets and surgical instruments of flint and bronze, as well as charms and amulets against the demons of disease.

The goddess of medicine was Ishtar, the Mother God, often called the weeping goddess because of her sympathy for suffering. She was invoked during childbirth and for women's diseases; but she was also goddess of love and war.

Gula was the goddess of death and resurrection and was often referred to as the "chief physician." She is shown receiving petitions from physicians about their patients; sometimes the supplicants wore masks of beasts to represent the demons of their disease. When the great King Assurbanipal was reigning in 800 BCE, he requested Gula to cure his son of "an insect-borne disease." Litanies were sung in the temples to call on her healing powers. Gula was also invoked to counter the female demon Lamashtu, who plagued women in childbirth.

Priestess-healers were always unmarried women and lived in the temples of Ishtar or Gula. They visited the sick in their homes to say prayers and to bury pomegranates and models of eyes under the floors in order to ward off evil spirits and statues of the goddess to invoke aid. Amulets have been found shaped like the head of a ram, inscribed with charms for safe pregnancy and labor. In the foundations of the Temple of Ishtar many rings, beads, charms, and amulets were buried, each inscribed with the name of the particular god or goddess associated with a disease and a prescription for the cure. The priestesses

5. *THE PAPYRUS EBERS*, CYRIL BRYAN (TRANS.), 1929, P.42.

studied their patients' dreams to help with their diagnoses, and prayers were said out loud in increasing volume to catch the attention of the goddess. A petition might be fairly simple; one example reads: "All the evil that is in thy body, may it be carried off with the water of thy body, the washings of thy hands, and may the river carry it down stream."

In the library of Assurbanipal (600 BCE) some eight hundred prescriptions on clay tablets have been found with instructions for treating a wide variety of ailments. Remedies include pinecone gum made into a soothing lotion, balsam, and the medicinal plant *Hyoscyamus niger* for headache, and castor oil cooked in beer for the eyes. A typical incantation runs:

O clear eye, O doubly clear eye,
O eye of clear sight!
O darkened eye, O doubly darkened eye,
O eye of darkened sight;
like a cup of sour wine thrown away,
Gula quicken the recovery, thy gift![6]

GODDESS MEDICINE IN THE MIDDLE AGES

Throughout the European Middle Ages "old wives" practiced medicine. These women used herbal medicine, ointments, collections of stones as amulets, and inscriptions as charms, which they sold to "believers." Most of them were itinerant and traveled from village to village holding clinics in the open air. They were regarded with a mixture of fear and awe. Their learning was probably passed down by oral tradition, usually from mother or grandmother to daughter. When their medicine was successful, it was called white magic; when it failed, black magic or sorcery. With a natural bent for healing,

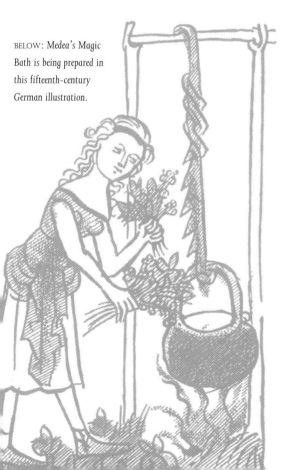

BELOW: *Medea's Magic Bath is being prepared in this fifteenth-century German illustration.*

---

6. *ASSYRIAN MEDICAL TEXTS*, R.C. THOMPSON, TEXTS, LONDON, 1924.

these women earned their living by using their secret remedies, which were usually a mixture of herbs and prayers, spells, and incantations.

Although physicians trained at the new universities tried to discredit these women, they were generally held in high esteem by the public. Some doctors even reported their successful cures: Arnold of Villanova saw an old wife cure a woman of septic sore throat with a plaster, and another cured a man suffering from hemorrhage with a secret remedy. Gilbert of England described a woman who had a potion called "burnt purple," which had occult powers and was reputed to cure smallpox. Most people accepted that medicine was made more potent if the doctor invoked supernatural powers, be they Christian or pagan. Although ostensibly Christian, Europe in the Middle Ages was pagan at heart, and in times of trouble people always reverted to the ancient religion. For this reason old wives were much sought after and their esoteric skills held in higher esteem than those of doctors.

The pagan religion was not as organized as the later Inquisitors would have us believe. There may have been gatherings or sabbats of witches, but the majority of wise women were simply following native customs. They respected the phases of the moon, were watchful for good or bad omens, and may have used some rudimentary astrology. Herbal lore was full of old wives' tales: plants with black berries, for instance, were to be avoided, whereas those with white berries were said to ward off evil spirits.

An account has survived of a leech working in Ireland whose house was open to the four winds and who had a stream of pure water flowing through his hall. This particular healer was a bonesetter and had several women helpers who actually set the bones. "Leech" is the name for such a healer, and many of them wrote down their recipes.

One, the Leech Book of Bald, which was written some time in the ninth century, has survived. In it Bald describes how certain plants were to be dug or cut at a particular phase of the moon, and how others were to be stabbed with a knife, while the collector prayed. The plants were washed in holy water from a church or magical spring, then spells were written on parchment and swallowed, or tied to the affected part. Often Christian saints were invoked, or paternosters or other prayers recited, but we can be sure this was no Christian ceremony, merely a practice designed to avoid the charge of witchcraft.

The following prayer was written down in England during the twelfth century, at the time of Hildegard. It is obviously a ritual chant, to be used when collecting and preparing plant medicine, but probably dates from a much earlier period.

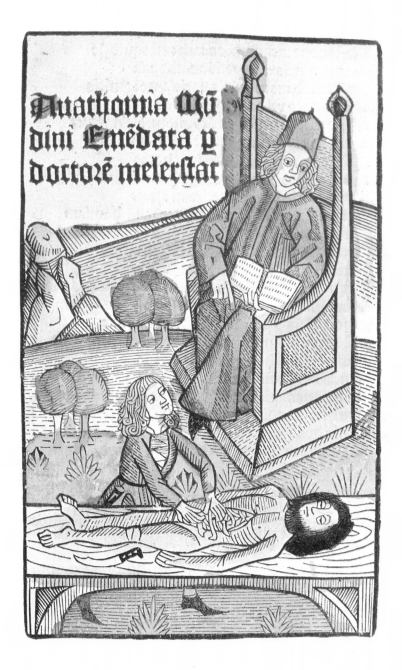

LEFT: *Leeches often had female helpers. This woodcut of 1493 shows "the anatomy lesson."*

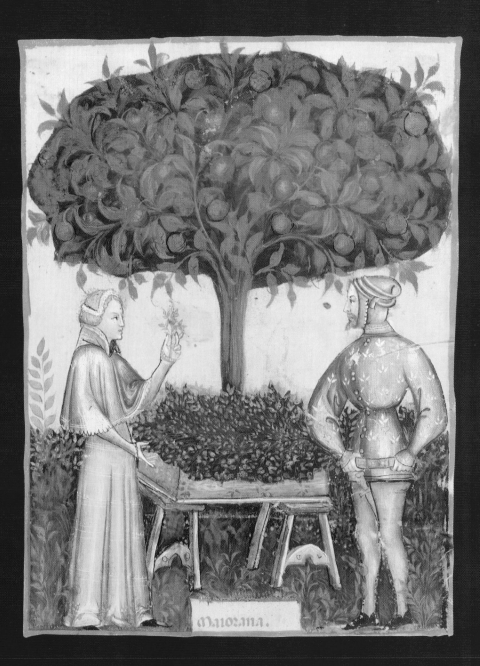

TWELFTH-CENTURY PRAYER

Earth, Divine Goddess, Mother Nature who generatest all things and bringest forth anew the sun, which thou hast given to all nations; guardian of sky and sea and of all gods and powers, and through thy power all nature falls silent and then sinks into sleep. And again thou bringest back the light and chasest away night and yet again thou coverest up most securely with thy shades. Thou dost contain infinite chaos, yea, and winds and showers and storms; thou sendest them out when thou wilt and causest the seas to roar; thou chasest away the sun and arousest the storm. Again when thou wilt thou sendest forth the joyest day and givest the nourishment of life with thy eternal surety; and when the soul departs to thee we return. Thou art indeed duly called Great Mother of the gods; thou conquerest by divine name. Thou art the source of the strength of nations and of gods, without thee nothing can be brought to perfection or be born; thou art great Queen of the gods. Goddess! I adore thee as divine; I call upon thy name; be pleased to grant that which I ask thee, so I shall give thanks to thee, goddess, with one faith.

Hear, I beseech thee, and be favorable to my prayer. Whatsoever herb thy power dost produce, give, I pray, with goodwill to all nations to save them and grant me this my medicine. Come to me with thy powers, and howsoever I may use them may they have good success and to whomsoever I may give them. Whatever thou dost grant it may prosper. To thee all things return. Those who rightly receive these herbs from me, do thou make them whole. Goddess, I beseech thee; I pray thee as a supplicant that by thy majesty thou grant this to me.

Now I make intercession to all ye powers and herbs and to your majesty, ye whom Earth parent of all hath produced and given as medicine of health to all nations and hath put majesty upon you, be, I pray you, the greatest help to the human race. This I pray and beseech from you, and be present here with your virtues, for she who created you hath herself promised that I may gather you in the goodwill of him on whom the art of medicine was bestowed, and grant for health's sake good medicine by grace of your powers. I pray grant me through your virtues that whatsoe'er is wrought by me through you may in all its powers have a good and speedy effect and good success, and that I may always be permitted with the favor of your majesty to gather you into my hands and glean your fruits. So shall I give thanks to you in the name of that majesty which ordained your birth.

LEFT: "Those who rightly receive these herbs from me, do thou make them whole." Marjory, in the Tacuinum Sanitatis.

MAMA LOLA:
A VOODOO HEALER

The Spirit is a wind. Everywhere I go, they go too...to protect me.

MAMA LOLA [7]

Mama Lola practices a healing tradition that has been passed down through three generations of her family, for she is a _mambo_ (priestess) in the Haitian Voodoo tradition. Mama Lola's mother was a famous mambo in Port-au-Prince. When Mama Lola was seven, she was bitten by a dog and disappeared for three days – she does not remember what happened or where she went. To her mother, this was a sign that the spirits had chosen Mama Lola as one of theirs. "My mother show me how to do good ... I remember every single thing she tell me, because that's in my family! My great-grandmother serve spirit, and my grandmother, then my mother, then me."[8]

Mama Lola "replaced" her mother, that is, she inherited her role. She was left her mother's altar, with its stones, pots, and other sacred items, and she also inherited her mother's diagnostic abilities. Her mother was known for her psychic abilities, but Mama Lola denies that she has this gift. She does admit to having "the gift of eyes,"

meaning that she "sees" the spirits: "I don't see light. I got the feel in my body. The blood goes up and my hair start to stand up if there is a spirit there that bothering somebody. I feel something inside that mean danger."[9]

Voodoo derives directly from the African slaves brought to Haiti. Because of the virtual isolation of that country, the religion is more authentic there than in any other Caribbean or Latin American country. Healing is the central core of this religion, although Mama Lola also works with problems concerning love, work, and family. In this respect she is a priest, social worker, psychotherapist, and doctor: "There is no Voodu ritual, small or large, individual or communal, which is not a healing rite."[10]

Moun feet pou mouri ("people are born to die") is a common Haitian saying. Suffering, _mize_, is expected and no one is exempt. Life is seen as suffering interspersed with times of luck or _chans_, and people who expect to live without suffering are regarded as naive. However, chans can be arranged, as the mambo works to ward off bad luck and attract good luck, which also brings health. Mama Lola heals by exercising, strengthening, and mending relationships among the living, the dead, and the spirits. Luck is controlled if this whole "family" is fed and cared for.

Many different types of problems can be helped by her treatment, but Mama Lola never pays

7. MAMA LOLA, A VODU PRIESTESS IN BROOKLYN, KAREN MCCARTHY BROWN, UNIVERSITY OF CALIFORNIA PRESS, BERKELEY, 1991, FRONTISPIECE. 8. IBID., PP.77–8. 9. IBID., P.354. 10. IBID., P.10.

much attention to the presenting problem or symptom, as it usually masks an underlying conflict. Invariably the root of the trouble is a relationship problem. But because these relationships involve the living, the dead, and the spirit world, diagnosis is by no means easy. First, she does a card reading to discover if the cause of the problem is "natural" or "unnatural." If it is natural, it is God-given, and there is nothing any healer can do about it, so Mama Lola sends these people away. Unlike the spirits, God cannot be bargained with, and what is made by him cannot be unmade by anyone. Resistance to cure is a sure sign that the malady is "unnatural," and there is hope that the spirits will intervene to solve the problem.

Voodoo healing works according to traditional wisdom. The mambos have a treasure-house of herbal knowledge, which they use to treat physical ailments. There are standard ritual forms

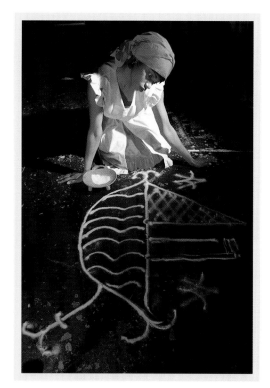

ABOVE: *Preparing a Voodoo symbol on the floor in advance of a healing ritual.*

of treatment, like baths, but the practitioner is allowed to invent as appropriate. When Mama Lola is unsure how to treat a patient, her mother sometimes appears in dreams and tells her which herb to mix with which flowers to effect the cure. The mambo therefore has to develop her intuition or *konesans*.

Mama Lola never refers to the people who visit her as patients, because in Voodoo, the one being healed has to be an active participant throughout the healing process, from the card reading – where the client may agree or disagree with the diagnosis – to the cure that has to be "worked," the prayers said daily, candles lit, perfume sprayed, medicine prepared, etc. The client is encouraged to build up his or her self-confidence to deal with the world as a poor black person. This is not to be confused with pride, which Mama Lola considers an American vice, from which no good can ever come. ❧

THE SANGOMA OF SOUTHERN AFRICA

The *sangoma*[11] are healers of southern Africa – generally women from the Nguni tribe – who are "chosen" by the ancestral spirit or *badimo* during puberty. This usually happens in the course of a severe illness, when the badimo comes to them in a dream. They then seek out an old sangoma for guidance and training. The individual cannot resist the "call" and, should she try to do so, will suffer from an illness that resembles a psychotic breakdown. The prophetic dreams vary in content but always involve a snake.

Their training involves divining, herbalism, and "sucking" (removing evil spirits by sucking them out of the body); it generally lasts two years and has to be paid for. In some cases sangoma specialize in a type of exorcism where they sing, dance, and play the drum, entering into a trance state. At puberty a special initiation ceremony is performed, which is held in secret.

Mrs. Jane M. is a sangoma and lives and practices from a round hut made of mud and cow dung, with a thatched roof. On the front is the sign "Jane is a doctor." She is about fifty and is married with children. Her first husband divorced her because she failed to have children, so she married again and treated herself for infertility, and now she has seven children.

Her mother was also a sangoma, and Jane believes she may have inherited some skills from her. Her powers were transmitted by a badimo who came to her when she was a young girl. He told her to go to the mountains, where she stayed for about a week. She remained in close contact with the badimo, who sent

LEFT: *A sangoma holding a traditional fetish in readiness for a ceremony.*

her the *theko* bird to keep her company. Now she always wears its feathers in her cap and often sings its song.

In order to receive training Jane first learned divination, and then spent three years learning from a herbalist. She paid one ox and one goat to the teacher. The herbalist also taught her how to "suck."

Jane now spends three to four months a year practicing in a nearby village: the rest of the year she works at home. She can collect her fees only if the patient recovers. She sees an average of two patients a day and spends about an hour with them. The treatment lasts from four to eight visits and is a mixture of healing and preventative medicine. She also protects houses from witchcraft and misfortune, cattle and crops from disease, and huts from lightning. She works with the nurse in the village clinic and will refer patients to her, particularly those with tuberculosis and venereal disease. The nurse visits Jane to watch her work and is learning her methods.

Jane wears a colorful skirt embroidered with the word "doctor" in ostrich eggshell and has a string of bones and pearls tied across her chest which are protection amulets. To make a diagnosis, divination is generally done by "casting the bones." The holy bones are kept in a small bag and are usually small pieces of ivory or antelope horn, jackal's teeth, goat vertebrae,

shells, or pieces of plastic or glass. The bag is made from goatskin, decorated with ostrich-shell pieces sewn on in a pattern.

The divination is performed in a group, with the diviner sitting on the ground and the patient and his family in a circle around him. The patient blows into the goatskin bag, and the diviner does the same and casts the bones. While she is reading them, the sangoma questions the patient about the disease and its possible cause. The bones reveal the reason for the disease, the prognosis, the treatment indicated, and whether the disease is due to impurity in the body or to witchcraft.

One woman patient came to Jane with pains all over her body and palpitations. During the divination it transpired that the young woman had been neglecting her old father. In the trance, the badimo became angry about her neglect of her filial duties and cast illness on her as punishment. Logically Jane recommended that the daughter look after her father better and bring him food every day. But a herbal treatment was also prescribed, which was smeared over the patient's body, and she was given a herbal medicine to drink. The patient recovered.

Jane believes that disease has increased in recent years due to the bad influence of the white man, but also that the badimo are unhappy about the way that people live in the villages and show their anger by causing disease. ❧

11. SEE FRANTS STANGARD, *TRADITIONAL MEDICINE IN BOTSWANA*, IPELEGENG PUBLISHERS, GABARONE, BOTSWANA, 1985.

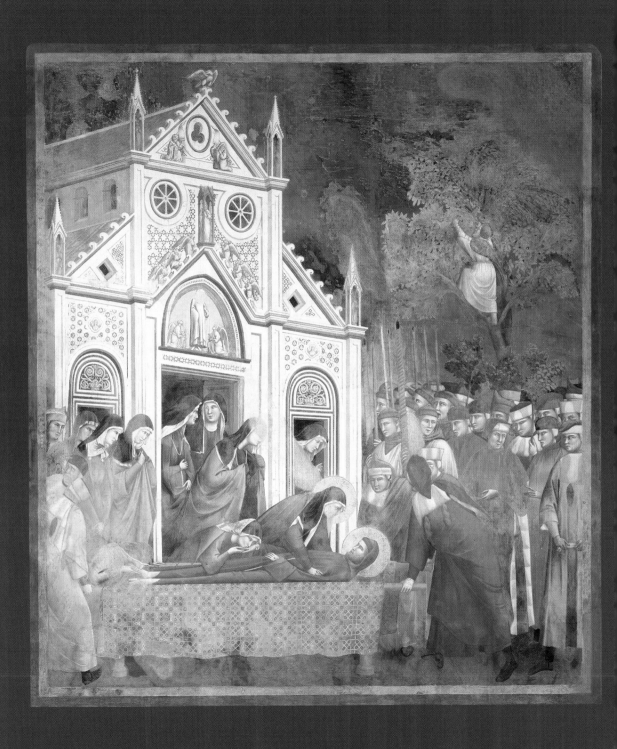

THE
HEALING CHURCH

~~~~~~~~~~~~~~~~~~~~~~~~~~~~~~~~~~~~~

HE early Christian Church allowed women an equal role. Jesus had several loyal women followers, among them Mary Magdalene, Susanna, Salome, Joanna, and Mary of Bethany, whom early Christian women took as their role models. The Acts of the Apostles detail the names of women who helped the new faith after Jesus's death.

In his parables, Jesus used the lives of both men and women as examples of faith, humility, and charity. He taught that the poor widow's gift was more valuable than the generous contributions of the rich, for hers was made with greater sacrifice (Mark 12:41–2). He used the metaphor of birth to describe his mission and promised that his followers would feel the joy a woman feels when she has given birth (John 16: 20–2).

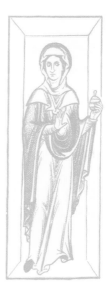

LEFT: *St. Mary Magdalene.*

LEFT: St. Clare embraces the body of St. Francis at the Convent of St. Damien by Giotto (c.1266–1337).

The Gnostic texts[1] are said to offer a more balanced view of the teachings of Christ than the Bible and to show his sympathy for, and value of, the feminine. An extraordinary poem found among the scrolls of the Nag Hammadi library runs like a Zen koan (or baffling mental puzzle):

1. SEE ELAINE PAGEL, *THE GNOSTIC GOSPELS*, RANDOM HOUSE, NEW YORK, 1979, AND BONNIE ANDERSON AND JUDITH ZISSNER, *A HISTORY OF THEIR OWN*, VOL. 1, PENGUIN, LONDON, 1988, PP.67–84.

I am the first and the last. I am the honored one and the scorned one. I am the whore and the holy one. I am the wife and the virgin. I am [the mother] and the daughter...I am knowledge and ignorance... I am shameless; I am ashamed. I am strength, and I am fear...I am foolish, and I am wise...I am godless, and I am one whose God is great.[2]

The early Christians followed these Gnostic teachings, but the more orthodox branch of the Church recoiled at the equality that the Gnostics permitted women, giving them a voice in the ministry. The first major Christian writer in Latin, Tertullian (190 CE), wrote, "Those women among heratics...They teach, they engage in discussion; they exorcise; they cure."[3]

The Christian followers of Valentin considered women equal to men, and some women acted as prophets, some as teachers, others as healers. But despite the teachings of Jesus and his moves to break the misogyny of Jewish culture by giving Mary Magdalene a role in his ministry, after 200 CE women were forced back into their subordinate role.

Besides healing, care for the sick was obligatory for the early Christians. They believed that at the Last Judgment Christ would say, "I was sick and you visited me" to those who were saved and, to the condemned, "I was sick and you didn't visit me."

Following this early tradition, the Church has been at the forefront of medical care for the poor. Early nuns opened clinics and rudimentary hospitals, which were the only form of health care available to the poor. In the Middle Ages nuns studied and copied medical texts as they became available, and many Christian women were physicians as well as scholars. Hildegard of Bingen wrote the earliest surviving scientific book by a woman.

Nuns continued their nursing role even though, after the thirteenth century, they were less concerned with acting as doctors. Instead they worked with Europe's untouchables, dying soldiers, lepers, and the insane. This role has continued to the present day.

In the nineteenth century various charismatic Christian movements came into being and the "laying on of hands" again became popular. Mary Baker Eddy (see p.40) can be seen as an extension of this tradition.

EARLY CHRISTIAN DEACONESSES

The first office created by the Church in Jerusalem was the diaconate. Deacons and deaconesses cared for the sick, but their ministry

2. "THE THUNDER: PERFECT MIND," 13.1616.25, *THE NAG HAMMADI LIBRARY*, J.ROBINSON (TRANS.), HARPERCOLLINS, NEW YORK, 1977, PP.271–4

3. *DE PRAECRIPTIONE HAERETICORUM*, TERTULLIAN, P.41.

was directed to the whole community, especially in times of epidemic. They were ordained by the laying on of hands. The first deaconess to be mentioned by name was Phoebe of Cenchrea, who lived around 60 CE. Paul refers to her in the Epistle to the Romans as a comforter to many, including himself.

With the closing of the pagan hospitals in 335 CE, when Constantine made Christianity the state religion, deaconesses began their healing work in earnest. They were mentioned as a recognized order in the councils of Nicea (325 CE) and Chalcedon (451 CE). They were ordained to minister to the needs of women in the congregation and to care for the sick and afflicted.

Olympias, born in 368 CE, became a deaconess at the age of twenty and worked among the poor and sick for the rest of her life. She had great powers of organization, and forty deaconesses were said to live under her rule. Placilla was the wife of the Emperor Theodosius and worked among the sick in Constantinople, where she "tended the bedridden with her own hands." Marcella was a young Roman widow, who put her palace at the disposal of the sick and needy. She died when the Goths plundered Rome in 410.

Fabiola became a Christian under the influence of Marcella and renounced her wealth to devote her life to minister to the sick and destitute. She built and opened the first Christian hospital in 390. It was called a *nosokomeion*, a house dedicated entirely to the sick. St. Jerome said of her, "How often did she wash the putrid matter from wounds another could not bear to look upon. With her own hands she prepared their food and moistened with water the parched lips of the dying." He claimed that "There was hardly an institution that had not benefited by her charity, hardly a bedridden patient in Rome who had not felt her care."[4]

Paula was another patrician woman born in Rome in 347. She was a friend of Fabiola and was instructed in the Christian faith by Marcella. She was a learned Hebrew scholar and helped St. Jerome translate some books of the Old Testament. She built a monastery in Bethlehem, founded a hospital in Jerusalem, and built hospices for the sick on the pilgrims' route to Bethlehem so that "none shall suffer on the road where Mary, mother of Christ, found no refuge but a stable." It is recorded that "she was piteous to them that were sick, and comforted and served them right humbly; and gave them largely of such food as they asked. She was oft by them that were sick, and she laid the pillows aright and in point; and she rubbed their feet, and boiled water to wash them."[5]

Eventually the order of deaconesses was suppressed, then abolished by the Synod of Orleans in 533, "by reason of the frailty of their sex."[6] ❧

---

4. *STORY OF THE GROWTH OF NURSING*, EDITH PAVEY, FABER & FABER, LONDON, 1938, P.103. **5.** IBID., P.104. **6.** IBID., P.105.

WOMEN, THE MONASTIC ORDER, AND HEALING

The early abbesses possessed considerable power, lands and influence in Britain. Abbess Mildred was given over 10,000 acres by King Egbert of Kent (664–73) to found a convent. Here she is said to have cured hundreds of parishioners with her medical skill. When she died, the dust from her tomb was said to have healing powers.

The Merovingian queen, Radegonde (525–87), founded a convent-hospital in Poitiers, France. She visited the sick, dressed their wounds, and bathed them. She opened a sanctuary for lepers in the palace precincts and personally supervised their care. She persuaded the king to let her take holy orders and eventually became abbess of her convent. She sold all her jewelry in order to finance the building of the hospital. Like Mildred, miracles were said to take place at her tomb.

There were two periods in European history when a great liberalization occurred in the Church, which allowed women a greater and more visible role in its offices. The first occurred in the twelfth and thirteenth centuries, and the second in the sixteenth and seventeenth centuries.

The Beguines were inspired by the teachings of St. Francis, and they responded to his call for chastity, austerity, and service to others in the popular enthusiasm of the thirteenth century.

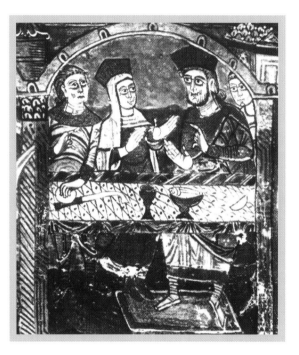

ABOVE: St. Radegonde, here seated at the table of her husband, King Clotaire, founded a convent-hospital and leper sanctuary in France.

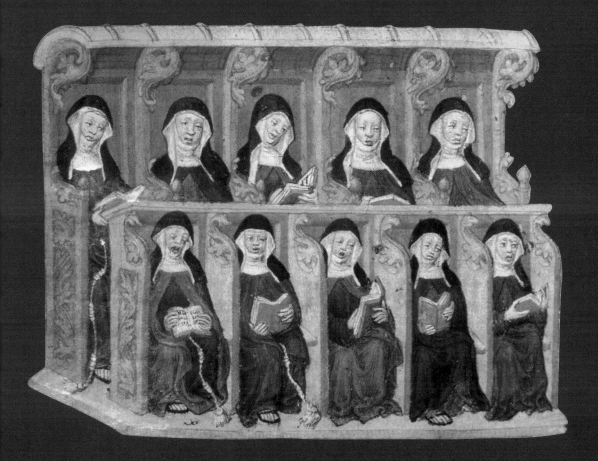

ABOVE: The Poor Clares, at service,
as depicted in Richard II's psalter.
They came to England in 1293.

They left their families, their marriages, and their material possessions and came together for a life of prayer and service. Their order was created in 1184 by a priest from Liège in Belgium. Lacking the funds to enter monastic life (women needed to bring a substantial dowry with them in order to become a bride of Christ), these women sold their belongings and created communal houses, or *béguinages*, in towns across northern Europe from the thirteenth to fifteenth centuries. They were resented by the orthodox Church, but were too numerous to be suppressed. By the fifteenth century it is estimated that there were 200,000 members of the Beguine order.

The hospital at Châlon-sur-Saône was started by the Beguines and became the home of the Sisters of St. Martha of Burgundy. Beguine hospitals flourished, although their property was confiscated by Protestants in Germany in the seventeenth century, and in France they survived only until the early seventeenth century. After the Battle of Waterloo in 1815, they again turned their buildings into hospitals and treated not only the soldiers but also the civilian population. They nursed the sick during the many cholera epidemics of the nineteenth century, both in their hospitals and in the homes of their patients. In times of flood, famine, and other natural disasters, they were on hand to give relief until other charities arrived. There are surviving Beguine orders at Ghent, Bruges, and Louvain in Belgium and at Amsterdam.

The Poor Clares, also called the Minoresses, were the second order of St. Francis. Clare, or Chiari Scifi, came from the noble family of Assisi, but ran away at seventeen to work with St. Francis in his community. Her piety attracted a large number of young women, who lived together in the olive groves of the hermitage of St. Damien. When St. Francis lay dying, Clare and her nuns nursed him. The Clares became an enclosed order and came to England in 1293, where they founded a nunnery in Aldgate, London, called the Minories.

Nearly all of the religious houses were closed during the Reformation and their property confiscated. After the French Revolution of 1789 several French branches moved to Canada and the United States. St. Mary's Hospital of Rochester, Minnesota, has always been run by Franciscan nursing sisters, and it is here that the famous Mayo brothers, founders of the world-renowned Mayo Clinic, performed their pioneering surgery.

The rule of the order of St. Clare reads, "The abbess is strictly bound to make compassionate and charitable provision for the sick according to the possibilities of the place...Because it is an obligation on all sisters to care for the sick as they would themselves wish to be cared for, if they were taken ill."[7]

---

7. *STORY OF THE GROWTH OF NURSING*, PP. 84–5

HILDEGARD OF BINGEN

1098–1179

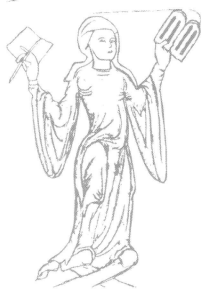

> Everywhere in creation there are mysterious healing forces, which no person can know unless they have been revealed by God.
>
> HILDEGARD

Hildegard of Bingen was unique in her time for the breadth and depth of her knowledge, ranging from science to music and theology, and for the respect afforded her by Popes and Emperors alike, who saw her as a true prophet.

The youngest of ten children, she was given into the care of the Church at the age of eight and was educated by the abbess, Jutta, under Benedictine rule. Hildegard succeeded Jutta as abbess in 1136, and founded her own abbey at Rupertsberg, Bingen, where she moved with eighteen nuns in 1147.

Her visions started when she was three years old, but she kept quiet about them until she fell ill around age forty and realized that this illness was the Holy Spirit insisting that she record them. For ten years she worked on her treatise *Liber Scivias* (Know the Ways of God), which was followed by *Liber Divinorum Operum* (The Book of Divine Works). In addition to these visionary books, Hildegard wrote several works on medicine and science, including one of the earliest surviving scientific books by a woman. In *Physica* (The Book of Simples) she describes over three hundred medicinal plants. In *Causae et Curae* she catalogues nearly fifty different diseases, speculating on their causes and recommending specific treatments. Her writings show that she was familiar with classical authors such as Pliny and Galen, as well as with contemporary medical texts from Salerno and other medical schools (see Trotula, p.86).

Hildegard wrote that disease stemmed from disruption of the body's equilibrium. She described the circulation of the blood hundreds of years before William Harvey discovered it in the seventeenth century, realized the connection between diabetes and sugar,

LEFT: *Hildegard of Bingen was a practical visionary.*

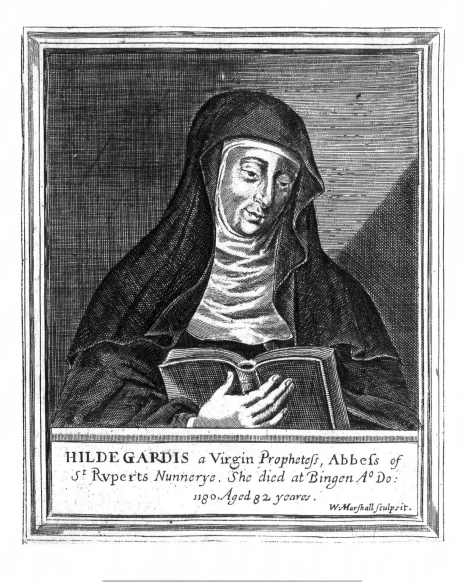

HILDEGARDIS a Virgin Prophete/s, Abbe/s of
St Rvperts Nunnerye. She died at Bingen Aº Do:
1180. Aged 82 yeares.

W. Marshall sculpsit.

ABOVE: Hildegard's writings showed a deep
understanding of the way the body works.

and understood the theory of contagion (not accepted by the medical profession until the nineteenth century). She wrote about the development of the female reproductive system, including descriptions of puberty and the prevalence of birth defects in very young or old mothers.

Her medical observations drew on popular medicine, which was used in the German clinic at Rupertsberg, and also on the long tradition of Benedictine medicine (Benedictines were physicians to the English royal family).

Hildegard viewed the human organism as a microcosm reflecting the macrocosm of the sacred world. She saw illness coming from sin, and both physical and mental pain from not respecting the Divine Will. She believed that humankind was intrinsically good and that our sins reflected the distortion of that good. She understood how mental states might give rise to physical illness: anger, for example, generates bile, which after a time produces harmful effects such as ulcers.

She believed that physical recovery happened only with the full cooperation of the whole person. The patient had to develop an ordered life and follow a sound diet – things not obtained through the use of medicine, but inspired by the spirit of balance and moderation. People needed to live in harmony with the elements in order to maintain internal harmony. But, in the final analysis, cure depended upon the will of God.

Hildegard called her image of health *viriditas* (greenness) or the "green lifeforce of the flesh."

When *blood and water decrease the eyes of a person too much because of age and sickness, this person should go to a green grassy garden yard and look at it for as long as the eyes are wet like from crying, because the green grass takes away whatever cloudiness was in the eyes and makes them clear and bright.*

CAUSAE ET CURAE, 209, 22FF

Hildegard practiced many forms of religious medicine: the laying on of hands, prayer, the use of blessed waters, amulets, and exorcism. The following is an incantation/exorcism for a woman sick with a gynecological disease:

Satan! *Leave the body of this woman,*
Allow the Holy Spirit to enter
Bad Spirits leave her body through putrid
vaginal discharges!
She has been freed![8]

---

8. *HISTORIA DE LA MEDICINA*, JAYNE & JAYNE, BARCELONA, 1993, P.93.

She also noticed the effect of the moon on body fluids and mental conditions. In *Liber Divinorum Operum* she wrote that human blood and the brain are swollen when the moon is full and that epilepsy often occurs when there is an eclipse of the moon.

She recommended the following to a sibyl, or seer, who had been hemorrhaging: "Place your trust in God. But around your chest and your navel set these words: 'In the name of Him who orders all things rightly; in the blood of Adam death arose; in the blood of Christ I command you, blood, to cease flowing.'" According to Hildegard (Vita, 3: 40, pl, 197:119 cd), it worked!

Hildegard argued that, by nature, women were colder than men and represented the body, while men represented the soul. She saw women as more sensitive to their physical environment, having the ethereal nature of Eve, and viewed a woman's body as a lyre. She believed that celibacy required a special vocation, and in *Causae et Curae* (60–2) she wrote about sexuality and conception using Galenic theory. She claimed that the four elements united to form a poisonous foam-semen, which remained poisonous until it was neutralized by the womb. She saw semen as cold and tainted, whereas menstrual blood was warm and pure – totally at odds with contemporary misogynist belief.

She believed that cold binds the menses, so for painful periods she recommended a gentle massage of the trunk and limbs to reverse the blood flow through the veins. She lists salves, herbal concoctions, potions, plasters, baths, and so forth; tansy, feverfew, and mullein were recommended for a cold womb. And in *Physica* Book 3 she recommended aspen leaves for babies:

> If any baby lying in its cradle is suffused and vexed with blood between the skin and flesh, so that it is greatly troubled, take new and recent leaves from the aspen and put them on a simple linen cloth and wrap the baby in the leaves and cloth and put him down to sleep, wrapping him up so he will sweat and extract the virtue from the leaves; and he will get well.

WOMEN SAINTS

St. Elizabeth of Hungary (1207–31), another thirteenth-century exemplar living outside of cloisters, displayed extremes of service and, during her short life, was regarded by the Church and lay people alike as a pious heroine. Her education was overseen by her aunt, Hedwig, Queen of Silesia, who herself built hospitals and leper asylums. Elizabeth studied medicine at the Wartburg castle near Eisenach and, after the death of her husband, Ludwig IV, she became a Franciscan tertiary, a member of a lay order that allowed religious women to live uncloistered lives. She founded the hospital of Marburg and worked selflessly with the sick and dying until her early death at twenty-four. Her fame quickly spread, and miracles were said to be performed at her shrine. She was made a saint only four years after her death.

Mechthild of Magdeburg (1212–83) was educated by Gertrude, the abbess at the German convent of Helfta. Mechthild was particularly interested in hygiene and practiced an early form of preventative medicine, centuries before its time. She believed in nourishing the body to do God's service and in the curative powers of sunlight, the natural world, and music.

In England, Abbess Euphemia of Wherwell, in Hampshire, was so powerful that she kept all the accumulated funds from her vast estates to build a hospital. One of her biographers said that she taught medicine and tended patients. One of her pupils, Agnes Ferrer, was sent to Constantinople in 1257 to care for the sick Crusaders. During the same century, Edina Rittle, who was working at St. Bartholomew's Hospital in London, was sent out to take charge of the great Pantocrator hospital built by Queen Alexis I in Constantinople.

In the seventeenth century bold Catholic women insisted on the right to live independent lives in the service of the sick and poor. St. Louise de Marillac le Gras (1591–1660), who was widowed early, became a follower of St. Vincent de Paul. He inspired the well-to-do women of Châtillon-en-Bresse to do something to ease the suffering and poverty caused by the religious wars and founded the Sisters of Charity, which became the principal nursing order of France. Women at the French courts like Madame de Miramion and Charlotte de Ligny used their own houses as orphanages and feeding centers. Louise de Marillac expanded and strengthened the movement, bringing in country women to help the "ladies."

From 1655 the Sisters of Charity functioned separately from the Ladies of Charity, with Louise de Marillac at their head. They nursed in institutions such as Saint-Denis in Paris and the battlefields of the Fronde and Calais. The sisters were disbanded during the revolution towards the end of the eighteenth century, only to be reconstituted by Napoleon in 1799. By the 1850s there were over 100,000 sisters, who nursed in prisons, military wards, and their own hospitals.

At the same time, the new Protestant churches also took on the care of the sick. Methodists, Baptists, and Quakers all took a part, founding many hospitals throughout the world and supplying them with female nursing staff. In 1823 Amalie Sievekig founded a sisterhood that

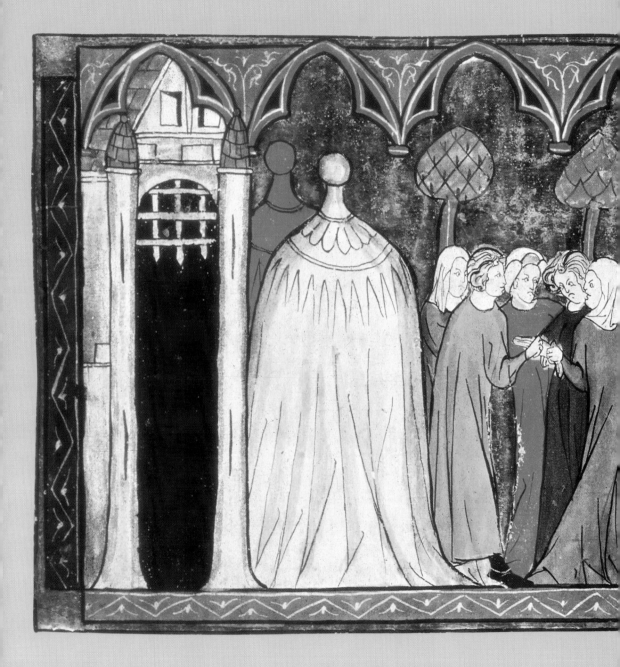

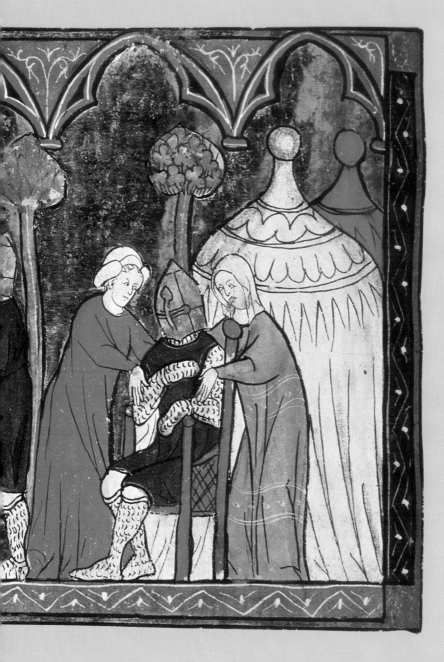

LEFT: Sick Crusaders were cared for by women such as *Agnes Ferrer*, who was sent to Constantinople in 1257.

nursed the victims of the great cholera epidemic in Hamburg. The first Protestant hospital was founded in Kaiserwerth in 1831, together with a diaconate of nurses, which soon had worldwide recognition. Florence Nightingale was one of those trained at Kaiserwerth.

Besides nursing work, the relics of saints and especially the power of prayer and the force of the Holy Spirit were crucial to Christian healing. The Virgin has appeared in special places throughout history, and these sites are ever after imbued with healing powers. Lourdes in France is an obvious example, but such shrines occur all over the world. The Virgin is gifted with powers of miraculous healing, and to this end incantations and prayers are said to her.

A variety of female saints are popularly believed to have healing gifts. St. Walburga was an eighth-century nun from Dorset, who traveled with her brothers to heathen Germany, eventually taking sole charge of the nunnery and monastery that they built together. Her name was often confused with the pagan Walborg, a Mother Earth figure. Walburga was a healer and was invoked by the Spanish against coughs and the plague. She was prayed to for eating disorders, and it is claimed that she cured a girl of a ravenous appetite by giving her three ears of corn.

St. Apolonia is the patron saint of tooth disease and dentists. She was martyred in Alexandria during the third century. Pagans tortured her by pulling all her teeth out, then built a huge bonfire and threatened to throw her in unless she renounced her faith. Instead, she threw herself into the fire and burned to death. She was venerated especially in Alexandria and Rome, but her cult also spread to Europe in the Middle Ages. It is still alive, and the following is an oration to her: "Saint Apolonia, here I am, poor sinner, my teeth hurt, please be reconciled with me and give me the rest I need for my body, so that I might forget this torment which is my toothache." ∾

MARY BAKER EDDY
1821–1910

Mary Baker Eddy, the founder of the Church of Christ, Scientist, suffered from ill health all her life, but was cured instantly by Phineas Quimby, a charismatic healer from Maine. She soon moved on to a system of healing based on the Bible's teaching and developed her own theories concerning the spiritual basis of sickness.

In 1866, while reading an account of one of Jesus's healings in the New Testament, Mary recovered from what she had considered to be the incurable effect of a serious accident. This prompted her to undertake several more years of intensive study, which gave her further valuable healing experiences.

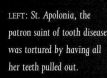

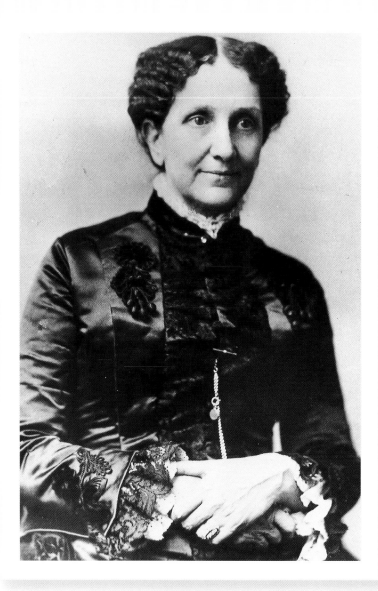

ABOVE: Mary Baker Eddy,
founder of the Church of Christ, Scientist.

In 1875 she published *Science and Health with Key to the Scriptures*, which she claimed was divinely inspired, and which forms the primary source for Christian Science beliefs. Four years later she founded the Church of Christ, Scientist, with the aim of reinstating "primitive Christianity and its lost element of healing." In 1881 she founded the Massachusetts Metaphysical College, where she taught her healing methods.

Mary Eddy believed that Jesus's healing works and his triumph over death demonstrate the defects and limits of the mortal state, which can be overcome as one "gains the mind of Christ." She saw matter as a limited form of human perception and viewed people as wholly individual and perfect, like the Creator, and thus incapable of suffering, sickness, and death.

In Christian Science healing rests on the belief that the patient may acquire a spark of the Divine Mind that Jesus possessed and so break through the material world of pain and suffering. Mary considered the regenerative process to be a long one, needing the Christian virtues of patience and humility.

The Christian Science practitioner is a self-trained, self-appointed healer. In the Church, practitioners come to healing through "inspiration" or a "calling," rather than by deciding they want to heal. At first they treat family ailments, then members of their Church may approach them. Over time, they build up a "reputation" as a healer. Each Wednesday night there is a meeting at which healings are discussed, and so the novices become known to the wider Church community as probationary practitioners. When they have sufficient experience and confidence, they apply to the Mother Church in Boston for permission to open a public healing practice. The requirements are that the probationer provides evidence of three healings, which must be diseases of a physical nature, such as heart disease, an infection, and so on. If they are accepted, the Mother Church lists the practitioner's name in the Church journal, which is read by members and the public alike. The practitioner may then open a clinic and start work as an approved Christian Science practitioner.

Mary Baker Eddy preached the spiritual equality of men and women, and women have always had a pivotal role in her Church. The vast majority of practitioners are women.

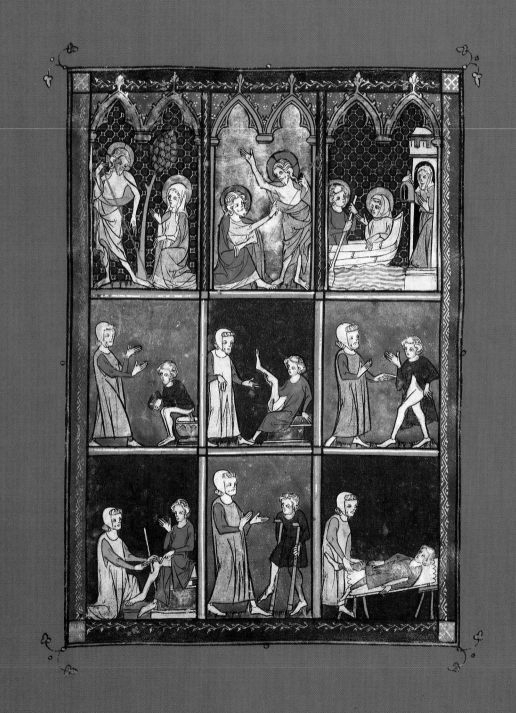

EDUCATION

*I*N the ancient world many Greek women were distinguished doctors, and from earliest times women doctors were found in Italy, Egypt, and Asia Minor. Theano was the wife of the philosopher, mathematician, and healer Pythagoras, and took charge of his academy after his death in 500 BCE. Pythagoras used music in his healing work, which Theano continued. In the works of the famous Greek physicians, Hippocrates, Galen, and Pliny, frequent references are made to the writings and practice of celebrated women doctors. Many of these treated women and children exclusively, while others practiced surgery and pharmacy, as well as general medicine. Deserving special mention is Metadora of Italy, whose manuscript on the diseases of women survives today in Florence.

After the fall of the Roman Empire, medical education was exclusively in the hands of the Church, and monasteries and convents were the only centers of learning and culture. Medicine became part of the curriculum for convent schools; no girl's education was complete unless she had an elementary knowledge of medicine and that part of surgery that deals with wounds. Women would be called on to cauterize wounds, stitch them, and set bones.

During the twelfth century there was a brief flowering of women's education, epitomized by Trotula in Italy and Hildegard in

LEFT: *Various medical ailments illustrated in the thirteenth-century Book of Surgery by Master Rogier de Salerne.*

Germany, both upper-class women. Hildegard used her mystical visions as a way into the scholastic world and was fortunate in having an educated monk to train her. We know less about Trotula, but she benefited from Italy's liberal attitudes towards women.

Italy was always in the vanguard of education and contained the best of Greco-Roman culture. Here, women enjoyed the rights and privileges accorded to men, and schools and universities were open to all, regardless of religion, sex, or race. Bologna, called *Legum Bolonia Mater* (Bologna, the Mother of Laws), has been witness to the blooming of female learning for thousands of years. The university there was in the forefront of women's education. Dorothea Bocchi was appointed professor of medicine and moral philosophy at Bologna in 1390, and she remained on the faculty for forty years.

After this time the only women who had access to education were those who had the financial resources to pay for tuition, nuns, and those whose husbands or fathers trained them. Formal education was available in the new universities but, with the exception of Italy, they were closed to women and non-Christians.

Despite these obstacles, women continued to study and write. Several fell foul of the Inquisition, which was suspicious of education in general and women's education in particular. But the majority of "irregular practitioners" working in towns and rural districts would probably have been illiterate, or just able to sign their name. Education for the "masses" only really became available in the nineteenth century, when philanthropists made wealthy by the Industrial Revolution opened schools and public libraries. With a few notable exceptions, university education remained closed to women until the twentieth century and, even then, access to medical education was restricted, and male students fought bitter campaigns to prevent women from studying. ✑

THE MEDICAL SCHOOL AT SAIS

From 4000 BCE a succession of women came to the throne in Egypt, and they allowed all their subjects – men and women – to study medicine. There were several royal medical schools – Pliny tells of one in Heliopolis (near modern Cairo) that had been in existence for hundreds of years when Moses and his wife Zipporah studied there. Graduates were given offices with good salaries and ran free dispensaries for the poor.

In the pyramids in the Valley of the Tombs of the Kings many pictures depict Egyptian life. In one of them is a portrait of Merit Ptah, *c.* 2500 BCE, the first female physician on record. Egyptian

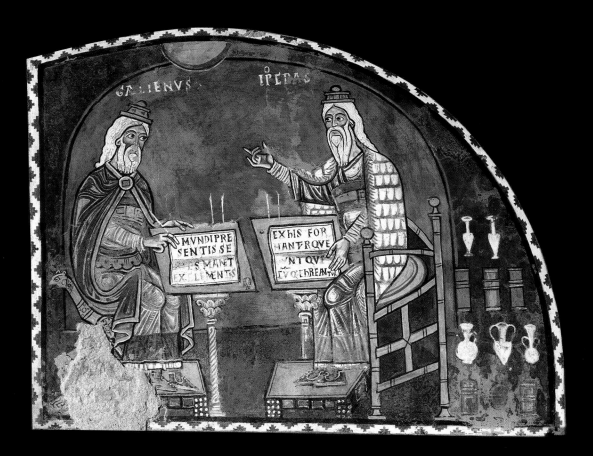

GALIENVS   O IPERAS

MVNDI PRE
SENTIS SE
ES MANT
EXELEMENTS

EX hIS FOR
MANTROVE
VNTQVE
TVQThREANTVR

ABOVE: The physicians Hippocrates and Galen
depicted in a thirteenth-century Italian fresco.

women shared equal status with men and were trained as physicians and surgeons. Women interested in obstetrics and gynecology trained at the medical temple at Sais. There an inscription reads: "I have studied at the women's school at Sais where the Divine Mothers have taught me how to cure diseases." Students would have used the famous medical papyrus, the *Kahun*, which gives detailed instructions on how to treat women's diseases. Female anatomy and surgery were taught, along with embalming. In the temple at Thebes is a picture of a slave girl doing an operation on the foot of a woman patient, dated around 1420 BCE. Helen of Troy was said to have studied medicine in Egypt and learned how to make the drink nepenthe, which she used to poison her enemies as well as to heal her friends, according to the dose. ✍

PROMINENT MEDICAL STUDENTS

Before the twelfth century, education took place either in religious establishments or privately, in a type of apprentice system. Women as well as men were educated in this way, and many female physicians were trained by their fathers or husbands. There was also a tradition of women following the profession of their deceased husbands – be they apothecaries, surgeons, or bonesetters. The Egyptians, Persians, and early Moslems allowed some noble women to study, but the first example we have of widespread women's eduation comes from Italy, and the University of Salerno.

Situated as it was on the southern Italian coast, Salerno had a transient population from Europe, the Far and Middle East. Newly translated medical classics were worked on at the university: Arabic, Greek, and Hebrew texts in particular. Medical students studied Arabic medicine, based on the teachings of Avicenna, and astrology, as well as the Seven Liberal Arts. Women were allowed to graduate in medicine and were known as the *Mulieres Salernitanae*; they also wrote various medical books and were professors at the university (see Trotula, p.86).

Abella was a Roman woman who wrote *De Atrabile et de Natura Seminis Humani* (concerning yellow bile and the human seed); another female doctor was Rebecca de Guarna, who wrote on fevers, urine, and embryology; and Mercuriade, a distinguished surgeon, published her thoughts on the treatment of fevers and embryology.

Another famous medical graduate from Salerno was Francesca, wife of Matteo de Romana of Salerno, who, after passing a strict examination in front of a panel of physicians and surgeons, was awarded a doctorate in surgery. The citation reads as follows:

Whereas laws permit women to practice medicine, and whereas, from the viewpoint of good morals, women are best adapted to the treatment of their own sex, we, after having received the oath of fidelity, permit the said Francesca to practice the said art of healing.[1]

The English universities of Oxford and Cambridge were closed to women, although women were able to study independently with teachers who had studied in Europe. However, the University of Montpellier in France allowed both women and non-Christians to study, but few doctors trained there. In 1272 there were only six qualified doctors in all Paris (its population being then 200,000) and five in London.

All these were priests, so men who did not want to be ordained had to practice without licenses. Records of the City of Paris in 1292 show thirty-eight unlicensed practitioners.

By the fourteenth century non-Christians were forbidden to practice medicine, which left "mainly barbers, quacks, and women who had no university education"[2] to care for the population. After the decimation caused by the Black Death of 1349, however, some women were allowed to study medicine in England.

By contrast, Italy still permitted women to enter university in the fifteenth century. Cassandra Fidelis of Venice and Padua wrote a book entitled Descientiarum Ordine, on the natural sciences and the treatment of disease, in 1484. And Beatrix Gallindo, educated in Italy, was elected professor of Latin and philosophy at Spain's University of Salamanca, although it is not known whether women were allowed to study there.

In Switzerland, Barabara von Roll (1502–71) was a learned physician who had studied medicine and botany and was often consulted by local doctors. She pioneered the treatment of mental illness, noticing the connection between physical and mental health, now called psychosomatic medicine. In Spain, Oliva Sabuco de Nantes Barrera (born 1562) wrote a number of philosophical books on the nature of humanity and the functions of the human body. She put forward the theory that the plague was an airborne illness and discussed the effect of pain on people and on the body. Her book New philosophy on the nature of man, unknown to ancient philosophers, which will improve human health and life, published in 1587, was denounced by the Spanish Inquisition and burnt – only two copies remain, both of which are badly defaced.

The first woman to receive a doctorate of medicine in Germany was Frau Dorothea Erxleben (born 1715).[3] Her father was a doctor,

1. COLLECTIO SALERNITANA, III, G. HENSCHEL, C. DAREMBERG AND S. DE RENZI, NAPLES, 1852–9, P.338, QUOTED IN H. J.MOZANS, WOMEN IN SCIENCE, D. APELTON & CO., NEW YORK, 1913, P.286. 2. A HISTORY OF WOMEN IN MEDICINE, KATE CAMPBELL HURD-MEAD, HADDAM PRESS, HADDAM, CONN., 1928, P.249. 3. THE MIND HAS NO SEX?, LONDA SCHIEBINGER,HARCORT UNIVERSITY PRESS, CAMBRIDGE, MASS., 1989, PP.250–7.

who allowed her to be educated at home with her brother. In 1740 Dorothea wrote to Frederick the Great, applying for permission to study at the new university at Halle; he gave her permission, but her fellow students and academics protested. One, Johann Rhetius, wrote a pamphlet pointing out that women were forbidden to practice medicine, so it was pointless to allow them to study the subject. Dorothea responded with a book entitled Inquiry into the causes preventing the female sex from studying, with an introduction by her father.

War broke out in Germany, so Dorothea was unable to graduate, but she did set up a medical practice. In 1753, when one of her patients died, three male doctors complained that "quacks" like Dorothea were ruining their practices, and that she shamelessly called herself a doctor. In response the authorities passed a law forbidding anyone who was not licensed to practice medicine. Dorothea replied that she was not a "quack," but had been taught medicine by her father and had written her doctoral dissertation, which she was prepared to defend. She also challenged any doctor who had not had a patient die to come forward.

Dorothea was sent notice that she would have to take her doctoral examination at Halle within three months. Because she was heavily pregnant, she appealed to Frederick the Great to take the exam the following year, and he agreed. Her case became a *cause célèbre*, and it was finally decided that she could be permitted to graduate and practice medicine, as this was not a public office (from which women were barred) but rather a profession.

Her doctoral thesis, Concerning Swift and Pleasant but for that Reason often Unsure Treatment of Sickness, argued that doctors often treated patients unnecessarily. She gave the example of irregular menses and went on to discuss the appropriate treatment in such a case. The dissertation and oral examination were conducted in Latin. In 1754 she was finally granted her degree.

Dorothea received so many requests for her dissertation that she translated it into German. She became the first woman to practice medicine legally in Germany, but her case was an exception, and the next woman did not graduate from Halle Medical School until 1901. Dorothea practiced medicine until her early death, aged forty-seven, in 1762.

By the nineteenth century the tide had begun to turn in Europe and a few determined women were able to get a university medical education. Germany was a pioneer in this respect. Regina Joseph von Siebold sat in on the lectures on physiology, obstetrics, and pediatrics at the medical college of Darmstadt and then set up in practice. She became highly respected and, in recognition, the University of Giessen awarded her a doctorate in medicine in 1819. Her daughter Carlotta studied with her mother and was admitted to the university of Göttingen, where she took a special interest in physiology, anatomy, and pathology. She was awarded her doctorate in obstetrics by that university.

Still in Germany, a French midwife, Madame Bovin, was awarded an honorary doctorate in medicine by the University of Marburg. Her book, *Memorial de l'Art des Acouchements*, recorded her work in obstetrics and her fine diagnostic skill, went into several editions, and was widely translated. Her doctorate, however, did not open the doors of the Royal Academy of Medicine, which remained closed to women.

In Italy, women continued to study at certain universities. One exceptional woman was Maria dalle Donne. She came from a peasant background, but her great intelligence was noticed and, after passing through several secondary schools, she went to the University of Bologna, where she graduated *maxima cum laude*, with a doctorate in medicine and philosophy. Her medical knowledge enabled her to take charge of the school for midwives in that city. When Napoleon passed through Bologna in 1802, he was so impressed by Maria's skill that he sponsored her for the Chair in Obstetrics at the university. She remained in that post until her death in 1842.

By the mid-nineteenth century more and more universities in Europe had opened their doors to female medical students. In Switzerland, the Universities of Zurich, Berne, and Geneva began to accept them. The first woman to obtain a medical degree in Zurich was a Russian, Nadejda Suslowa, in 1867. In Russia itself, the Medical Academy of St. Petersburg awarded a degree to Madame Kaschewarow in 1869 – the first Russian woman to obtain this honor. Her fellow students carried her triumphantly through the hall after the degree ceremony. France's first woman graduate was Elizabeth Garrett of England, who could not study in her own country. And in 1879, Mary Putnam graduated in medicine in New York. The last country to allow women to graduate in medicine was England, which admitted women only after a long and bitter struggle. ✍

MARIA MONTESSORI
1870–1952

Maria Montessori was the first woman to obtain a doctorate in medicine in modern Italy, from the University of Rome in 1896. From 1899 to 1901 she was director of the State Orthophrenic School of Rome, and during the period 1896 to 1906 she held the Chair of Hygiene at the Women's College in Rome. From 1900 to 1907 she lectured in pedagogy at the university, and from 1904 to 1907

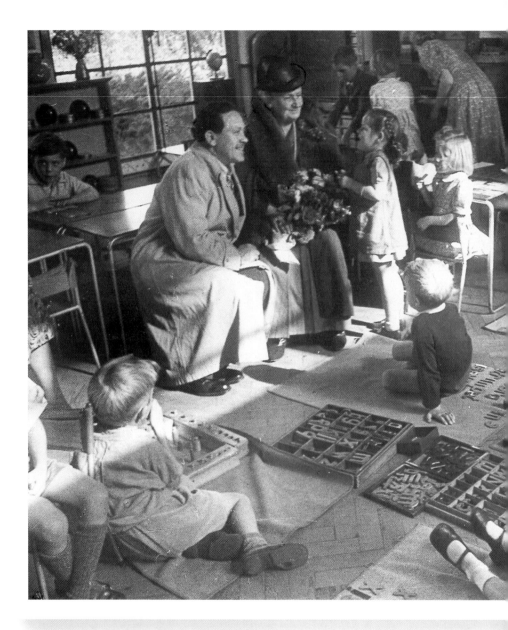

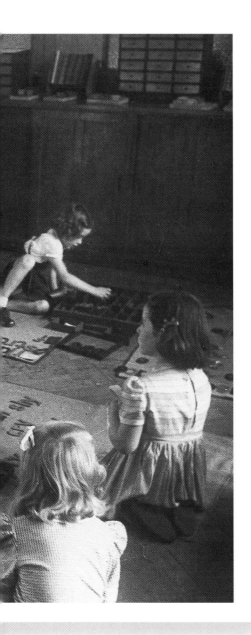

LEFT: Maria Montessori visits one of her schools,
which allowed children to develop at their own pace.

held the Chair of Anthropology. During these years she continued her studies in philosophy, psychology, and education. She worked intensively in the psychiatric clinic of the Rome medical school, where she came into contact with children suffering from growth and emotional development problems.

Maria came to the conclusion that these children were capable of reaching a far higher level of development than was generally expected of them. She therefore resigned from the university and from her medical practice to run a school for mentally retarded children.

In 1907 she opened La Casa dei Bambini in San Lorenzo, a poor area of Rome. It was a home for children from the ages of three to six, the sons of poor laborers. The work, undertaken by trained assistants, involved directing through creative channels the physical and psychic energies of these normal but disadvantaged children. Maria taught by giving children simple materials, believing that even the most unsettled children could develop their creative powers. Her theories proved correct and the children thrived in the liberal environment.

Working from a strongly spiritual bias, Maria Montessori encouraged the child's natural emotional and spiritual development through instructive play. There are now Montessori schools worldwide. ∾

MARIE STOPES
1 8 8 0 – 1 9 5 8

Marie Stopes opened the first birth-control clinic in the British Empire on March 21, 1921, in a modest house in Holloway, London.[4] The venture was financed by herself and her husband. Previously, birth control had been a taboo subject – only prostitutes used contraceptives, as respectable married women were supposed to welcome each new child. Defending her cause, the radical George Bernard Shaw wrote ironically to her, "reproduction is a shocking subject, and there's an end to it."

And one poor London woman put her own case forward:

> *Oh, there's enough babies in Poplar, if it's babies you want...We don't know how to stop 'em do we? I wish you'd tell us...I've heard of that woman, Marie Stopes is it? and I'm going to write to her. I've had my four a lot too quick, and I want a rest from having babies.[5]*

Some recent feminist researchers have attacked Marie Stopes for her eugenic policies (not too many working-class babies needed), but they have failed to take into account the acute need among poor women of her day to reduce the number of pregnancies.[6] During a rally held to

---

4. SEE DEBORAH COHEN, *PRIVATE LIVES AND PUBLIC SPACES: MARIE STOPES – THE MOTHERS' CLINIC AND THE PRACTICE OF CONTRACEPTION, HISTORY WORKSHOP JOURNAL* 35, 1993, PP.93–116. 5. IBID., P.97. 6. SOME FEMINISTS FELT THAT SHE WAS SINGLING OUT POOR WOMEN FOR CONTRACEPTIVE ADVICE SO THAT NOT TOO MANY POOR PEOPLE WOULD BE BORN. I DO NOT BELIEVE THIS WAS HER INTENTION – SHE WAS SIMPLY RESPONDING TO THE WOMEN'S NEED TO REDUCE THEIR FAMILY SIZE.

raise funds, Dr. Jane Hawthorne spoke out in favor of Marie's clinic:

[One]...of my cases is that of a woman who has had fifteen children, five of whom are living. At the clinic one day she said she was afraid that she was going to be the mother of another... I asked if her husband was not anxious to help in any way. She looked rather surprised and all she said was: "When I tell him there is another baby coming, he invariably kicks me down stairs."[7]

Marie's overwhelming priority was the health and happiness of her women patients and ensuring that they could have healthy children when they wanted them. She set out to redeem birth control from its association with prostitution and to link it with respectability and responsibility. She gave it the title "constructive birth control." The clinic was designed to be as welcoming as possible, with a light, airy waiting room and friendly female staff.

In 1925 the clinic moved to Whitfield Street, in central

RIGHT: *The young Marie Stopes wih cat.*

7. *THE TRIAL OF MARIE STOPES*, MURIEL BOX (ED.), FEMINA BOOKS, LONDON, 1984, P.24.

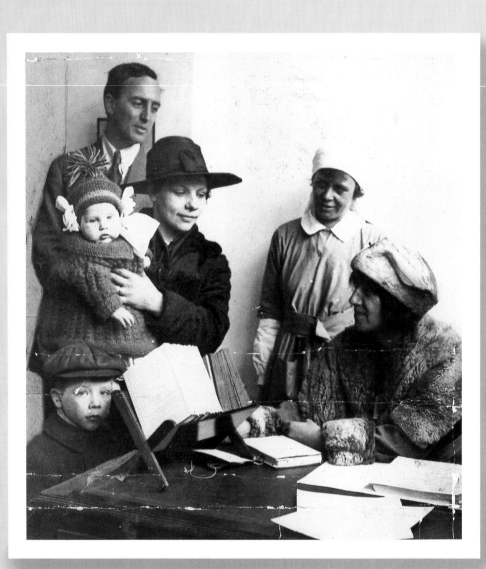

ABOVE: *Marie Stopes offers advice to a client
at her clinic, 1923.*

London, where it remains to this day. Marie decided that midwives and not physicians should give advice, and she always hired married midwives, with a preference for those who had children. This woman-to-woman contact was part of her philosophy, for she wanted "...a kind heart there to listen."[8] A client consulted only one midwife, who interviewed her, examined her, and taught her how to use a birth-control device. Marie put great emphasis on the midwives' character, and they had to be sympathetic, kind, and persistent, in order to gain trust but also to reach the correct diagnosis. Most women would be frightened by the experience and the aim was to put them at their ease:

> Everything has been planned and thought out with the idea of making the clinic a happy, helpful place...where gentle patient midwives and doctors, themselves married women, understand the problems and are ready quietly to spend all the time necessary to help and instruct inquirers.[9]

On the first day of the London Mothers' Clinic a queue of women waited outside, attracted by a poster announcing free birth control. When the doors were opened, the midwives waited for the patients to appear, but nothing happened, as the women were too frightened to enter the clinic.

The receptionist, Mrs. Richardson, had to go out and lead them in by the hand. This shyness was to continue, women being afraid and ashamed to be seeking contraceptive advice. Many patients had other gynecological problems but would not take them to a male doctor. The midwives, often working-class women themselves, could sympathize with their patients.

Because of the taboo women felt about touching their own bodies, midwives often spent hours with patients encouraging them to insert a contraceptive cap. The midwives needed endless patience, and many of them had long experience of working in mother-and-baby clinics. If a woman could not pay, Marie Stopes insisted that she be given free contraceptives, although some of the health workers felt that this was setting a bad example.

The aim of the clinic was not only to give birth-control advice but also to give marriage guidance, psychosexual counseling, and fertility treatment. By 1929 the London Mothers' Clinic had advised 10,000 patients, and Marie opened other clinics in five regions of the United Kingdom and two "caravan clinics," which traveled to rural areas in England and Wales. The clinics survive to this day and were used as models when family-planning clinics were opened on the National Health Service during the 1960s.

8. COHEN, OP. CIT., P. 99. 9. IBID., P.99.

RADIANT MOTHERHOOD

A BOOK FOR THOSE WHO ARE CREATING THE FUTURE

Coming parenthood and the adjustments of married lovers are treated in the light of beauty and joy springing from true understanding

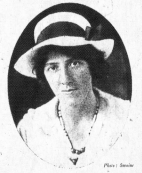

Photo: Swaine

By MARIE STOPES, D.Sc., Ph.D.

AUTHOR OF "MARRIED LOVE"

CLOTH, **246** PAGES, **6/-** NET

ABOVE: Radiant Motherhood, published in 1920, followed Marie Stopes' bestselling manual Married Love in 1918.

THE STRUGGLE FOR MEDICAL EDUCATION IN NINETEENTH-CENTURY AMERICA AND BRITAIN

Elizabeth Blackwell (1821–1910) enrolled as a medical student at Geneva College, New York, and graduated with an M.D. in 1849. She also studied obstetrics and midwifery in Paris at La Maternité. She undertook a lecture tour throughout England and struck up a lifelong friendship with Florence Nightingale.

In 1857 she joined forces with her sister Emily and Marie Zakrzewska to open the New York Infirmary for Women and Children (see p.111). In 1868 she founded the Women's Medical College of the New York Infirmary and took the Chair of Hygiene.

Encouraged by Elizabeth's success at Geneva, Harriot Hunt, who had been practicing medicine for twelve years, applied to Harvard Medical School in 1847. But her application was rejected. Geneva turned its back on women a few years later when it refused Emily, Elizabeth's sister, entry. Emily was eventually accepted by Rush College, Chicago, but the State Medical Society censured Rush for admitting women, and Emily was not admitted for her second year. She finally graduated from Cleveland Medical College in 1854.

The Blackwell sisters' decision to open a medical school stemmed from the belief that other schools for women offered an inferior education. They established entrance examinations long before the mainstream medical schools did so, and the course had a three-year program with longer than average terms and ample opportunity for clinical training. This placed the Women's Medical College well ahead of the typical medical school of its day – Harvard, for instance, did not establish a three-year curriculum until 1871. The school also had an independent board of examiners in order to maintain standards.

The next breakthrough came in the 1870s when the Universities of Michigan, Boston, Syracuse, Iowa, and California agreed to accept women. Dr. Elizabeth Mosher remembered "the day we read in the Boston papers that the University of Michigan had opened its doors to women in all departments. We five young women joined hands and danced around the table. We all went to that college and graduated there with a degree of M.D."[10]

It was the admission of women to the prestigious Johns Hopkins School that seemed to signal victory. A group of women launched a campaign to endow the university medical school on the condition that it admit women; $500,000 was raised – an offer too good to refuse – and three women were admitted to the medical course in 1893.

---

10. "PIONEER WORK" IN *OPENING THE MEDICAL PROFESSION TO WOMEN*, DR. ELIZABETH BLACKWELL, NEW INTRODUCTION BY DR. MARY ROTH WALSH, SCHOCKEN BOOKS, NEW YORK, P.IX.

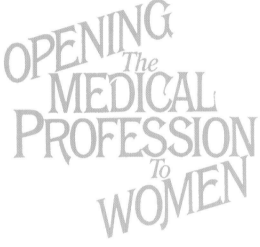

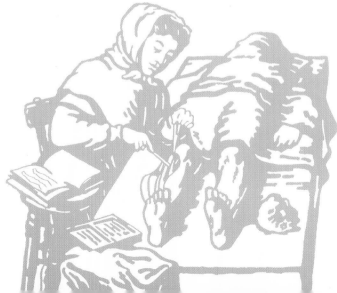

In 1899 the Women's Medical College of the New York Infirmary closed. It had graduated 364 women physicians in thirty-one years. Dr. Emily Blackwell said, "We had held open the doors for women until broader gates had swung wide for their admission."[11]

But by the first decade of the twentieth century such optimism was premature and retrenchment was apace. One reason for this was the great success of women doctors – failure was forgivable, but success was not. The result was the establishment of a quota system, limiting women's places to five per cent.

No real progress was made until 1970, when the Women's Equity Action League filed a complaint against every medical school in the United States. This and other suits, in conjunction with the federal government's Affirmative Action program, led to a sharp increase in the number of women medical students.

LEFT: *The front cover of Elizabeth Blackwell's book.*

11. IBID., P.XI.

Sophia Jex-Blake and five other women began medical studies at Edinburgh University in 1869, but a riot in 1870 made their case notorious, and they were denied the right to graduate after completing their studies. They eventually went on to graduate from Berne, in Switzerland.

In 1874 a group of women, headed by Sophia Jex-Blake and Elizabeth Garrett-Anderson, opened the London School of Medicine for Women, with rigorous academic standards and tutors who were women already qualified in medicine. The medical hierarchy attacked the school and threatened to blackball any male member who gave classes there. No teaching hospital would allow women to conduct clinical practice, and none of the nineteen examining bodies would give women the recognition they needed in order to be on the medical register. This state of affairs continued for the next three years.

In 1877 the Royal Free Hospital finally allowed women access to its facilities in a five-year experiment. In February, 1878, it was accepted by the Secretary of State as one of the medical schools qualifying for the University of London exams, and in 1910 the Royal College of Physicians and Surgeons finally opened its examinations to women. Dublin accepted women in the early 1880s, while Edinburgh, Aberdeen, Glasgow, and St. Andrews followed suit by opening to women in 1895. ✎

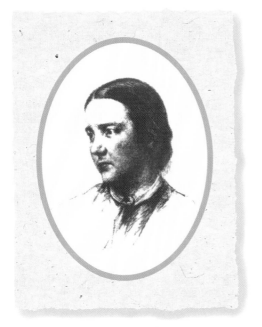

ABOVE: *Sophia Jex-Blake, one of the early women medical graduates and a founder of the London School of Medicine for Women, now the Royal Free Hospital.*

In Britain Elizabeth Garrett-Anderson (1836–1917) became the second woman on the medical register in 1866 (Elizabeth Blackwell joined in 1858). She had been unable to study in England, though, and had graduated from the University of Zurich in 1865.

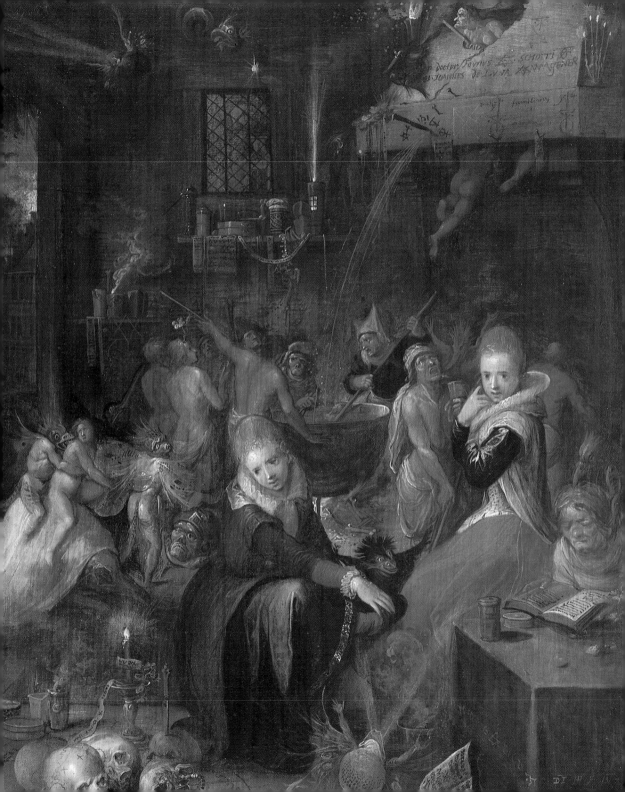

PERSECUTION

~~~~~~~~~~~~~~~~~~~~~~~~~~~~~~

*W*OMEN have been persecuted for practicing medicine for hundreds of years. Throughout the centuries women have been doctors, but so complete was the suppression of their history, that by the nineteenth century the received wisdom was that the combination woman/doctor was an impossibility. The process of excluding women from the medical profession was a long and bloody one, culminating in the witch-hunts in the seventeenth century.

Women were denied education and then blamed for being illiterate; were refused access to universities and then judged for not having licenses; when they used their natural "psychic" abilities, they were condemned as witches. Yet despite these tremendous obstacles, they continued to practice medicine, often more successfully than their male colleagues.

Most women doctors overcame the tremendous odds because they felt "called" to practice medicine, or they had seen a female member of their family or a woman friend die unnecessarily because she would not allow a male doctor to examine her. Many male doctors were in any case incredibly ignorant about female physiology.

One of the first recorded women to fight this prejudice was Agnodice, an Athenian woman doctor in ancient Greece. She

LEFT: *Witches' Sabbath by Frans Francken.*

studied medicine, disguised as a man, under the famous physician Herophilus (c. 300 BCE) at the medical school in Alexandria. Women were forbidden on pain of death to practice medicine in Greece, but, driven by a call to ease the suffering of her fellow women, Agnodice practiced secretly, until she was denounced one day by a jealous colleague. Hauled before the courts, she was tried, found guilty, and sentenced to death. Her women patients, hearing of her fate, marched on the court house. They threatened to commit mass suicide unless she was freed and pardoned. Many of the women were wives and sisters of the judges and other powerful men in Athens. The judges were forced to back down, and Agnodice was given a pardon. From that time on, gentlewomen (not slaves or foreigners) were allowed to practice medicine.

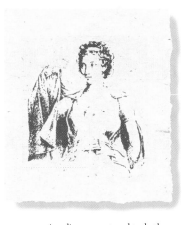

ABOVE: *Agnodice was sentenced to death for practicing medicine in ancient Greece.*

But the Christian Church, especially, was opposed to women having a role outside the home, and over the centuries, women's sphere of influence was gradually reduced. It took a long time, especially in rural areas where pagan beliefs persisted and women were seen as natural healers. Women continued to treat sick members of their families, but as soon as they tried to set up in some way as a "professional," the full weight of the law and the displeasure of the Church crashed down upon them.

The Industrial Revolution and its radical effects on the world offered women a chance to escape from the home, and education became a possibility for women who could afford it and whose family permitted it. The first wave of feminism at the start of the twentieth century saw a rush of women doctors, which was reduced to a trickle in the war years, and only the cultural revolution of the 1960s fully opened the door of the medical profession to women. ᴥ

EXCLUSION BY LICENSE

Between the twelfth and thirteenth centuries, secular law prohibited the clergy from bloodletting (4th Lateran Council), but lots of empirics (nonuniversity-trained doctors) – both men and women – continued to practice. Many, indeed, were trained by physicians, but as the majority were illiterate, they had little opportunity to expand their practices.

In the twelfth century the *Regimen Sanitatis Salernitanum* (the famous code of health of Salerno, concerning hygiene and medicine) became the medical bible of the Middle Ages. And Arabic medicine, considerably more advanced, became widely disseminated; the Arab and Persian physicians Avicenna (980–1037) and Rhazes (850–923) were especially widely copied, once translations were made available through the University of Salerno (see p.48). From the Arabs came myrrh, cinnamon, nutmeg, senna, cloves, and musk, and they also made distilled waters, which became a great favorite with apothecaries.

In 1220 the faculty of medicine at the University of Paris forbade all but bachelors from the practice of medicine, but little notice was taken of this. Montpellier made similar laws, which were also ignored. The first licensed woman doctor in Germany is believed to have lived in Frankfurt in 1288. Many physicians were Jewish women from Moorish Spain, where they had trained with Arab physicians.

In the fourteenth and fifteenth centuries women could practice in Florence, Venice, Naples, and Rome. One medical license of the fourteenth century read, "since, then, the law permitted women to exercise the profession of physicians and since, besides, due regard being had to purity of morals, women are better suited for the treatment of women's diseases."[1]

Beginning in the thirteenth century, Italian towns licensed doctors; German and French towns followed suit in the fourteenth century; English and Spanish in the sixteenth. By the beginning of the seventeenth century, to be a doctor, a surgeon, an apothecary, or a midwife required some sort of examination and licensing. England exemplifies how gradually women were excluded from medicine. In 1390 an examination was required for masters of medicine in London. University training was necessary for success but women were barred from the universities. Men denied women access to education and then prohibited their membership of professional organizations.

In the fifteenth century a petition was made to the English Parliament not to allow any unlicensed men or women to practice medicine. It was presented by John Mirfield of St. Bartholomews, London:

Worthless and presumptuous women usurp this profession to themselves and abuse it; who possessing neither natural ability nor professional knowledge, make the greatest possible mistakes (thanks to their stupidity) and very often kill their patients: for they work without wisdom and from no certain foundations, but in a casual fashion.[2]

1. *MEDIAEVAL MEDICINE*, J.J. WALSH, LONDON, 1930, P.158. 2. *JOHANNES DE MIRFIELD OF ST. BARTHOLOMEWS, SMITHFIELD, HIS LIFE AND WORKS*, SIR P. HORTON-SMITH HARTLEY (ED.), CAMBRIDGE, 1936, P.122.

In 1540 Henry VIII authorized a separate London surgeons' guild, to which women were forbidden membership. The same happened in Salisbury in 1614. Surgery became the exclusive practice of the free brothers, and the guild forbade outsiders: "no woman, or any other, shall take or meddle with any cure of chirurgery."[3]

After 1614 it became difficult for a woman to get a license for surgery, as the "barber-surgeon charter" came into force. To secure a license, the candidate had to be examined by the Bishop of London, who was more interested in heresy and witchcraft than in the candidate's professional qualifications. In 1617, when apothecaries were separated from grocers, a woman could not even obtain a license to compound medicine. And if women did break the law, they were liable to prosecution and imprisonment, as happened to surgeon Prudence Ludford in 1683.[4] Others were pardoned, such as Margaret Waltham, a "female practitioner" at Dorchester, who was dismissed by the court although it was recorded that she ministered to a child with a rupture.[5]

In the fifteenth and sixteenth centuries, in towns like Lille, Paris, Regensburg, and Strasburg, midwives had to appear before the local bishop to take an oath and before the secular authorities as well. By this time the licensing authorities were more concerned about when she should call in the male professionals, than with her own

expertise and testaments to her character. They also wanted to be sure that she practiced no other branch of medicine. "Midwives, under threat of corporal punishment, shall absolutely desist from extracting the placenta forcibly. In the event that it does not soon appear spontaneously, they must without hesitation request and seek the counsel of a licensing physician."[6]

In Paris midwives had a higher status and were examined by a physician, two surgeons, and two senior midwives. Their professional oath included the following: "If I foresee any danger I will call Physicians or Surgeons or women who are more experienced in the matter, and would not do anything without their advice or help."[7]

Midwives were especially suspect as the general persecution of "witches" gathered pace from the fifteenth to seventeenth centuries. The textbook for the Inquisition, *Maleus Maleficarum*, contained two chapters about midwives, claiming that many were witches who would kill the child in the womb and offer its soul to the devil. This was reflected in midwives' oaths. A Parisian midwifery oath of 1560 included the sentence: "I will not use any superstitious or illegal means, either in words or signs, nor any other way, and will do nothing in revenge or in personal anger."[8]

Increasingly, medicine became regulated and controlled. At the top of the professional hierarchy were the university-educated

3. *A HISTORY OF WOMEN IN MEDICINE*, K.C. HURD-MEAD, HADDAM PRESS, HADDAM, CONN., 1938, P.399. **4.** IBID., P.400. **5.** IBID., P 400. **6.** MIDWIFERY ORDINANCE, CITY OF NUREMBERG, FIFTEENTH CENTURY, QUOTED IN *MIDWIVES AND PHYSICIANS DURING THE RENAISSANCE*, THOMAS G.BENEDEK, *BULLETIN HISTORY OF MEDICINE*, 51, 1977, P.555. **7.** IBID., P.558. **8.** IBID., P.561.

physicians; below them came apothecaries and barber-surgeons, who were trained in the apprentice system or, if women, by husbands or fathers; and at the bottom came the "untrained" midwife and herbalist, who would learn from other practitioners, or whose knowledge was passed down from generation to generation. ✍

THE WITCH CRAZE

The *Malleus Maleficarum* was written in 1486 by two Jesuit priests, Heinrich Krämer and Jacob Sprenger, and became the witch-hunter's bible. It followed a papal bull issued by Innocent IV in May 1252, which called for: "a terrible measure against heretics in Italy, authorizing the seizing of their goods, imprisonment and torture, and, on conviction, death."[9]

Originally intended to stamp out heresy – that is, opposition to the established Church – witch-hunting became over the five centuries that it continued more "woman-hunting" than anything else. By the seventeenth century, ninety per cent of condemned witches were women. A veritable reign of terror swept through Europe, and millions of women died. Evidence was gathered on the basis of heresay and gossip; neighbor denounced neighbor; old scores were settled; and feuds over land were enacted in these courts. The courts were ecclesiastical and had "special powers." Torture was mandatory and involved sleep deprivation, public stripping to search for "witches' marks," which might be moles or birth marks, thumbscrews, gang rape, ducking, and the rack. Torture was officially sanctioned in 1257 and remained a legal recourse of the Church until 1816. Under these conditions anyone confessed to anything. Fredrich von Spee, a Jesuit who confessed the accused women, wrote, "Take the Capuchins, the Jesuits, all the religious orders, and torture them – they will confess. If some deny, repeat it a few times – they will confess. Should a few still be obstinate, exorcise them, shave them, only keep on torturing – they will give in."[10]

Soon whole villages were accusing one another, and in one town in Germany there was said to be only one woman left alive. Financial considerations were important. The Inquisition would confiscate the worldly goods of the accused and might exhume the dead, try them, and then appropriate their wealth. The accused were also charged for their own torture. In Scotland, for example, they were charged six shillings and eight pennies for branding on the cheek. The Church became extremely rich during these years.

Particularly targeted were independent women, spinsters, and widows, or those who did not conform to the low status afforded them by the Church. Women healers and midwives came

9. *WITCHCRAFT IN THE MIDDLE AGES*, J.B. RUSSELL, CORNELL UNIVERSITY, ITHACA, NEW YORK, 1972, P.155. **10.** *OCCULT SCIENCES IN THE RENAISSANCE*, WAYNE SHUMAKER, UNIVERSITY OF CALIFORNIA, BERKELEY, 1972, P.62.

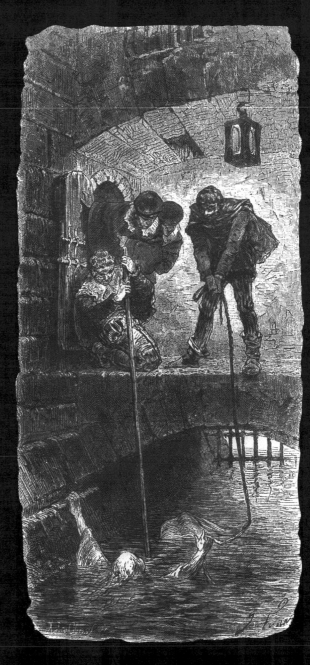

RIGHT: *A witch being ducked — wise women and midwives were often accused of witchcraft.*

into these categories and were hounded by the Inquisition. Wyer, writing in *The Dark World of Witches*, said that, "Ignorant and clumsy physicians blame all sickness which they are unable to cure or which they have treated wrongly, on witchery."[11]

It is doubtful whether the majority of women so accused were really witches, pagans, or satanists. The evidence taken under torture is highly questionable and would tax the credulity of any unbiased person. Many were probably natural psychics, clairvoyants, and what we would today call spiritual or charismatic healers. They were in fact carrying on the traditions of the early Christians in using spirit to heal.

The motivation was probably misogynist. By the sixteenth century an exclusively male medical profession was trying to establish a monopoly. What could have been more irritating than to have competition from barely literate women, who seemed to have a "natural" gift for healing? ∾

JACOBA FELICE

Jacoba Felice de Almania[12] (born 1280) was brought before the courts in Paris in 1322 charged with illegally practicing medicine, for she had no license: "The said Jacoba visited the sick folk, laboring under severe illness in Paris and the suburbs, examining their urine, touching, feeling and holding their pulses, body and limbs."[13]

The main witness for the prosecution was John of Padua, who had been surgeon to the King of France. He argued that there had been a law in operation for over sixty years that forbade the practice of medicine without a license. He claimed that Jacoba's crime was very serious, as an unlicensed woman might kill her patient. The penalties were prohibition and excommunication, which were applied with the full approval of the bishop's court in Paris as well as that of the kings of France.

Jacoba was a famous practitioner, and in her defense she brought many witnesses who testified to her success with patients. They stated that they had heard of her through word of mouth; that she had behaved as most physicians did in her examinations; that she refused payment until the patient was cured; and that no one had asked for her qualifications.

One witness, John of St. Omer, testified that he had been cured of an illness – Jacoba had visited him several times and had done more for him than any other other physicians called to treat him. Yvo Tueleu, related how she had been suffering from a fever and had been visited by several physicians, none of whom had been able to cure her. Jacoba, however, had given her a glass of very clear liquid, which had cured her of the fever.[14]

---

11. *THE DARK WORLD OF WITCHES*, ERIC MAPLE, A.S. BARNES & CO., N. J., 1964, P.49. **12** JACOBA IS ALSO CALLED JAQUELINE FELICIE DE ALMANIA, A CHRISTIAN VERSION OF HER NAME. BUT IT IS LIKELY THAT SHE WAS A JEW, AS THERE WERE MANY FAMOUS AND SKILLED FEMALE JEWISH DOCTORS IN EUROPE AT THAT TIME. **13.** *CHARTER OF UNIVERSITY OF PARIS*, II, PP.257-8. **14.** IBID., P.259.

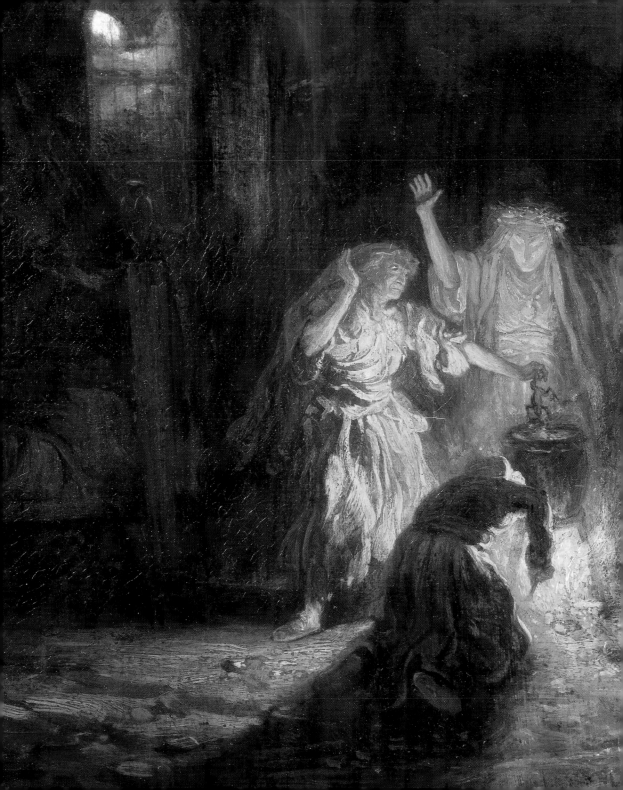

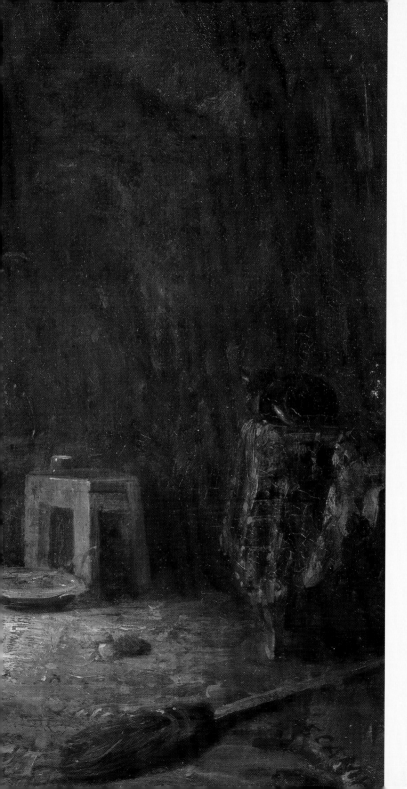

LEFT: The Witches
in Macbeth by
*Alexandre Gabriel
Decamps* (1803–60).

Also cited in her defense was the fact that there were many, many unlicensed practitioners in Paris. Jacoba also supported the argument that women should be given the opportunity to consult another woman, should they choose to do so:

It is better and more seemly that a wise woman learned in the art should visit the sick woman and inquire into the secrets of her nature and her hidden parts, than a man should do so, for whom it is not lawful to see and to seek out the aforesaid parts, not to feel with his hands, the breasts, belly and feet of women. And a woman before now would allow herself to die, rather than reveal the secrets of her infirmities to a man.[15]

Her defense also questioned the legality of the law, which, they claimed, had been invoked by the medical faculty of the University of Paris and had no legal validity. They declared that the statute could not be binding, as it went contrary to the public good, for women wanted to be seen by female physicians and it was only right that they should do so.

Despite the evidence, Jacoba was found guilty and excommunicated. The court decided that: "Her plea that she cured many sick persons whom the aforesaid masters could not cure, ought not to stand and is frivolous, since it is certain that a man approved in the aforesaid art could cure the sick better than any woman."[16]

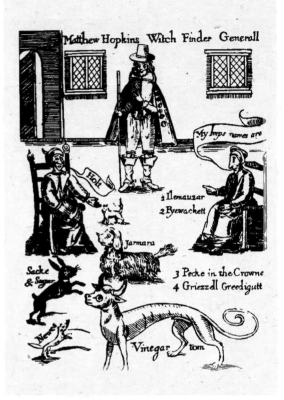

ABOVE: *Matthew Hopkins, the famous "Witch-Finder General" of mid-seventeenth-century England, investigates two witches and their familiars.*

15. *CHARTER OF UNIVERSITY OF PARIS, PP.257–8.* **16.** IBID.

Her real crime had been not malpractice, but the jealousy she engendered among her male colleagues. ☙

PERSECUTION IN SEVENTEENTH-CENTURY NEW ENGLAND

Jane Hawkins, midwife of Boston, was not formally accused of witchcraft.[17] However, she was banished from Massachusetts after one of her patients, Mary Dyer, gave birth to a deformed fetus, or "monster." Her enemies claimed that this was a punishment on both from God.

> Jane Hawkins, the wife of Richard Hawkins, had liberty till the beginning of the third month...in the meantime she is not to meddle in surgery, or physic, drinks, plasters, or oils, nor to question matters of religion...
>
> Jane Hawkins is enjoined to depart away tomorrow morning, and not to return again hither, upon pain of severe whipping.[18]

Hawkins and Dyer were friends and supporters of Anne Hutchinson, the charismatic spiritual leader of a sect known as the Antinomians. Hutchinson was also present at the birth, and several months later her own pregnancy ended in spontaneous abortion. It was claimed that this was another monstrous birth and implied that devilish things were afoot. Anne Hutchinson was banished in 1638. Mary Dyer left the colony but returned in 1660, when she was executed by the government. Anne Hutchinson returned to Massachusetts but was banished for a second time in 1641.

The governor of the colony, John Winthrop, kept a journal of the "monster-birth and its discovery" in which he connected Mrs. Hawkins's religious "heresy" with both women's sexuality and witchcraft:

> The midwife...used to give young women oil of mandrakes and other stuff to cause conception; and she grew into great suspicion to be a witch, for it was credibly reported that, when she gave any medicines (for she practiced physic), she would ask the party, if she did believe...these...gave cause of suspicion of witchcraft, for it was certainly known [she] had much familiarity with the devil...[19]

Margaret Jones of Charleston, Massachusetts, was a "cunning woman" who also performed midwifery and had a reputation for being able to foretell the future. She was tried and executed on June 15, 1648. John Winthrop described how she was found to have been "practicing physic...she would used to tell such as would not make use of her physic, that they would never be

---

17. SEE DAVID D. HALL (ED.), *WITCH-HUNTING IN SEVENTEENTH-CENTURY NEW ENGLAND*, NORTHEASTERN UNIVERSITY PRESS, BOSTON, PP.19–23, 230–51; AND CAROL F. KARLSEN, *THE DEVIL IN THE SHAPE OF A WOMAN*, W.W.NORTON & CO., NEW YORK, PP.14–21. **18.** THE MINISTER, *MASS. BAY RECS.*, 1, PP.224, 329. **19.** ANNE HUTCHINSON, *WINTHROP'S JOURNAL*, 1, P.268; 2, P.8.

healed, and accordingly their diseases and hurts continued, with relapse against the ordinary course, beyond the apprehension of all physicians and surgeons."[20]

Early in 1680 Elizabeth Morse's neighbors complained that she was a witch. The depositions show that she was actually a healer. She was brought to trial in Boston in May, 1680, found guilty, and the governor sentenced her to execution, which was later reprieved. The evidence of a neighbor, Jane Sewall, described Elizabeth as a "healing and destroying witch."

Elizabeth worked as a midwife and one Elizabeth Titcomb described how her own sister, suffering a long, hard labor, called for Goodwife Morse who, when she arrived, managed "a present speedy delivery of the woman."[21]

There is no satisfactory evidence to suggest that the women who were involved in birth defects were anything other than lay healers who had the misfortune to preside over births that ended in tragedy. Several of them were commited Christians, but they belonged to the Antinomian sect, which was seen as threatening the *status quo*. ᐸᕀ

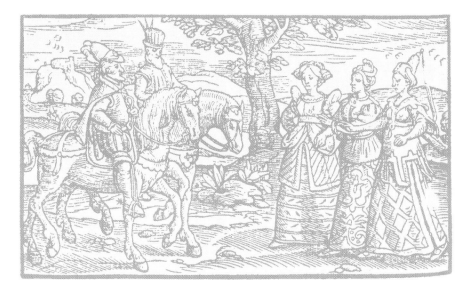

ABOVE: *Accusers were not above using the skills of witches when it suited them.*

20. *WINTHROP'S JOURNAL*, 2, PP.344–5. **21.** *MASS. BAY RECS.*, 1, P.340.

WOMEN HEALERS PERSECUTED IN SCOTLAND

At the same time, women healers in Scotland were being persecuted for practicing medicine.[22] In the case of Bessie Paine, indicted for the "sin of witchcraft" in 1671, the connection with her healing work is clear: "Cuthbert Brown of Craigend his first wyffe being sick He sent for Bessie Paine who befoir shoe was spoken to Concerning the nature of the Disease told that Agnes Rowan had witched her And yre-eftir shoe [hereafter she] went and cured her." What the verdict was is not recorded.

In 1699 Margaret Provost was also accused of witchcraft. The Laird of Suddie heard gossip that Margaret was a witch. He went with his servants and "pulled down her house about her ears" and, within a day or two, one of the servants swelled up "as bigg as two men." They challenged Margaret, who replied that if they would rebuild her house the man would be cured, and "the gardener became better."[23]

William Perkins, a Scottish minister and leading witch-hunter, made the following statement about women healers: "[the] good witch was more a monster than the bad." He claimed that the "blessing witch" (she who healed), although she did no actual harm and did "much good," was to be censured because "he [sic] hath renounced God...and hath bound himself by other laws to the service of the enemies of God and his Church, death is his portion."

The accusers were not above using the "witch's" healing skills, however: Alison Peirson of Byrehill was renowned as a skillful healer, and the Archbishop of St. Andrews called for her. His ailments did not respond to the ministering of orthodox medicine, and it is believed they were more "psychosomatic" than physical. Alison, however, cured him. Not only did the clergyman refuse to pay her bill, but he had her arrested and executed for witchcraft.

A similar fate awaited Gilly Duncan, a young servant girl of Edinburgh, who had a great reputation as a healer. People traveled large distances to consult her, but her master, David Seaton, heard of her fame and decided that her skill was diabolic. He tortured her by applying thumbscrews and jerking her head with a rope. She confessed to being a witch and was turned over to the authorities, who continued the torture until she "confessed" about her accomplices. These women, known as the "witches of North Berwick," were hanged in 1592.[24]

King James IV of Scotland (James I of England) believed that supernatural forces threatened his life. He commissioned the first translation of the Bible into English, rendering the famous Exodus 22:18 as "thou shalt not

22. *A SOURCE BOOK OF SCOTTISH WITCHCRAFT*, CHRISTINE LARNER, CHRISTOPHER HYDE LEE AND HUGH MCLACHLAN, UNIVERSITY OF GLASGOW, 1977, REF: JC26/38, CASE NO.599. **23.** *THE BOYDS OF TRCHRIGG*, LARNER ET AL., IBID., CASE NO. 3064. **24.** *WOMAN AS HEALER*, JEAN ACHTERBERG, RIDER, LONDON, 1990, P.90, UNSOURCED.

suffer a witch to live," although the word *kashaph* is best translated as "poisoner." He thus condemned many hundreds of thousands of women to a terrible death.

The Protestant Church was perhaps even sterner with women healers than the Catholic, and the numbers of women accused of witchcraft rose after the Reformation. Again, there is no evidence that these women were in any way connected with pagan beliefs, although as country women they would have been learned in old wives' tales. ❧

NATIVE AMERICAN PRIESTESS

Dhyani Ywahoo is a priestcraft holder of the Ani Gadoah Clan, Tsalagi (Cherokee) nation. She claims a lineage of twenty-seven generations, who have been "keepers of the sacred fire and crystals." She is founder and director of the Sunray Meditation Society in Vermont and has traveled widely throughout the world, including in India, Tibet, and Turkey, sharing her healing practices with other traditional healers and learning from them. Dhyani works with healing crystals, meditation, and chanting. She sees illness as a result of wrong thinking, and of being out of step with the "Great Spirit." She was taught that the most important thing was the power of thought and the voice and to look beyond surface ugliness to find the inner beauty that everything, and everyone, possesses.

As a Native American,[25] Dhyani (whose name means a gift of light and fire for the people) has experienced prejudice at first hand. She tells the story of being called a "red nigger"[26] when she went into town with her sister and grandfather. He was also a healer and used the incident to teach Dhyani about the difference between "whole and compartmentalized people." He told her not to show anger or be upset, but to pray for these ignorant people, for, in his words, "they do not know their hearts."[27] Her grandfather went on to explain that such people want to experience the Indians' inner peace (Dhyani refers to herself as an Indian, not a Native American) but do not know how. Racists have lost contact with their higher selves. Some weeks later this same person came to Dhyani's grandfather about a problem that she had, and he gladly healed her.

Dhyani says that she works to transmute negative energies, like rage and jealousy: "Energies change through transformation and non-attachment. I don't resonate to anything which is not whole."[28]

In the Cherokee healing tradition both men and women are healers, although Dhyani admits that the way they heal is often quite different. Men tend to remove the illness from a sick person's body, whereas women "change the

25. SEE BOBETTE PERRONE, HENRIETTA STOCKEL AND VICTORIA KRUEGER, *MEDICINE WOMEN, CURANDERAS AND WOMEN DOCTORS*, UNIVERSITY OF OKLAHOMA PRESS, NORMAN, 1989, PP.57–82. **26.** IBID., P.66. **27.** IBID. **28.** IBID., P.67

light" in the body. Men also heal by frightening or shocking the sickness out of the patient, whereas women nurture and render the patient childlike, vulnerable, innocent.

Within the tribe, women are valued as different but equal. They have their own healing circles, which a man may join if he wishes; in the men's healing circles they always invoke the feminine principle. Women are seen as the glue that cements the tribe together. Woman's role as "mother" is central to this. Women who have had children have a gap in their light aura, which means they are always giving energy to their children, and to every living thing, through that gap. The medicine woman has to learn to close that gap, which is very difficult, and is why women are so respected in Cherokee society.

Dhyani sees women's anger in speaking out about the rape of the land and the awful consequences of technology as an urge to return to the male-female balance that she grew up with in the Cherokee nation, which she describes as matrilineal. She gives this blessing:

"May you be surrounded ever in the light of wisdom and joy, and may...[it]bring many women again to the certainty of their gifts, and may men...realize the mother within, and may we all realize ourselves in the circle of light."[29]

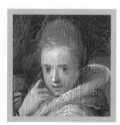

29. IBID., P.82.

զասացեալ աղկատարակ գամ ու . ե
լցկոյնտաբեէ երկնէ եկեալ . եւ ի այ
ամինքն յերկնէ եւ րս . զօրեն աս յեան
եւնիզատե . եւասե զասատակարա
աս ձեկեա զնսընզատական հայ . եւ քրաս
հեկեաց զնոսա ծառամեն . եւասաց ՃՃ
եւ որել չեք այն ձայնա աս աս արհաննէ ծառամեն :

MIDWIVES

*I*N many cultures birth is seen as a magical event and birth attendants, midwives, are often associated with the numinous, the sacred. In earliest times, midwives worked from temples, in Sumeria, Egypt, Africa, the Aztec and Inca kingdoms. Throughout the world noble women had their labor managed by the priestesses of their religion. Peasant women relied on neighbors, friends, and family, and the midwives' skills were passed on from woman to woman. Young girls watched births and learned by observation how to manage labor. Skilled midwives could turn the baby in the womb, and Caesareans were performed by Egyptian midwives thousands of years ago.

Because so many women died in childbed, most of the writings on childbirth contain magical formulas to invoke goddesses who might protect the mother. The more sophisticated the society, the more problems women seem to have had. Writing in the sixteenth century, churchmen recorded the indigenous women of the Caribbean delivering their children by themselves, quickly and seemingly without much pain, and then carrying on with their lives. But the wealth of petitions and charms suggests that even in undeveloped cultures, birth was never a straightforward procedure.

Midwives, then, learned through a hands-on approach and generally had had several children themselves. It was not until the

LEFT: *The Birth of Alexander, from a fourteenth-century Armenian copy of the fifth-century* Romance of Alexander.

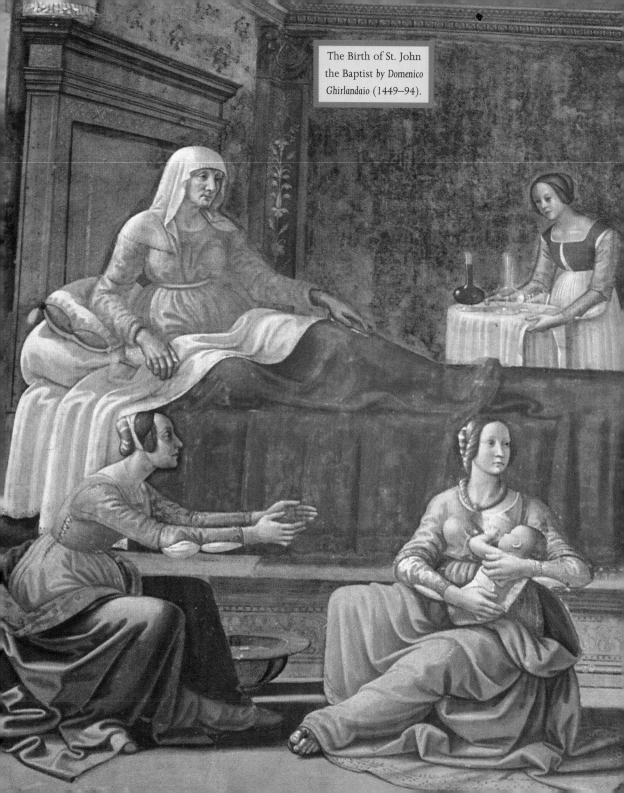

The Birth of St. John the Baptist *by Domenico Ghirlandaio (1449–94).*

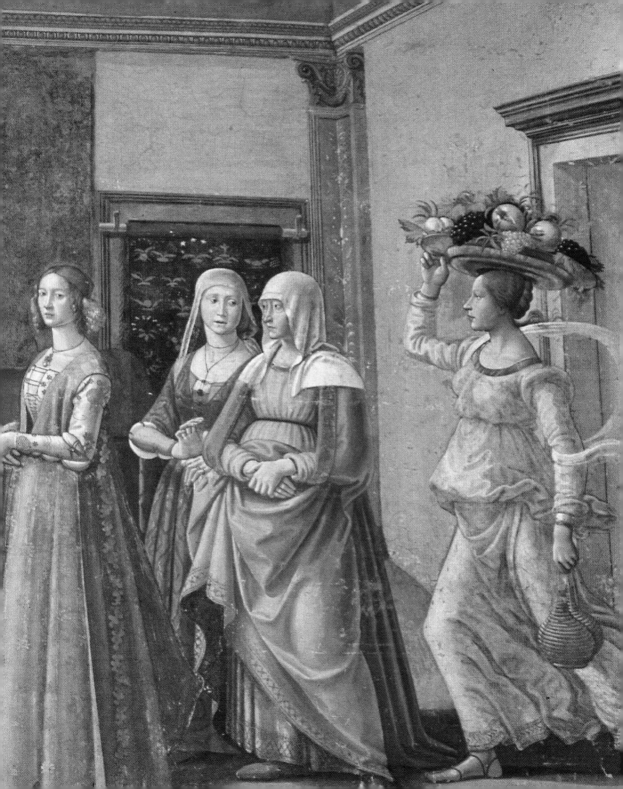

combined forces of the medical profession and monotheistic religion interfered that men had anything whatever to do with the process.

With the establishment of a male-run medical profession, first in Europe and then throughout the world, there has been a battle for control of childbirth. In some countries midwifery was virtually nonexistent, or until recently midwives practiced illegally (much of Europe and the United States). In others they were tolerated but were seen as low in status, semiliterate, and generally rather backward. In Britain midwives are today making something of a comeback as women begin to demand "natural childbirth" and the right to a home delivery. Recent studies have shown that deliveries involving midwives and home births are statistically safer than hospital obstetric births, confounding what has become the received wisdom about midwifery skills.

Within more traditional societies, men are seen as irrelevant to the birth process, and male doctors will only be used as a last resort. Indeed, in rural communities today, especially in Africa and South America, men are forbidden in the delivery room. In Africa, midwives usually live in the community in which they practice, speak the local language, and understand local customs and health beliefs. Midwifery is characterized by this practical approach, with birthing skills passed on from generation to generation. Because of its low

status, little was written about midwifery in the developing world before the last century, but we can assume traditional birth practices have changed very little.[1]

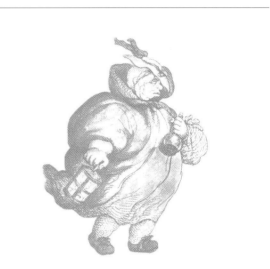

ABOVE: *A midwife going to a labor, as envisaged by Thomas Rowlandson (1756–1827).*

THE MIDWIFERY TRADITION

Until recently, European women generally gave birth at home, helped by their female neighbors and family members. Male doctors were called only in dire emergencies, because they knew little about female anatomy and for reasons of expense, since they charged fees only the rich could afford.

In the second century CE the Roman doctor Soranus described the ideal midwife:

---

1. SEE BONNIE ANDERSON AND JUDITH ZISSNER, *A HISTORY OF THEIR OWN*, VOL. 1, PENGUIN, LONDON, 1988, PP.39–44, 106–50, 294–6.

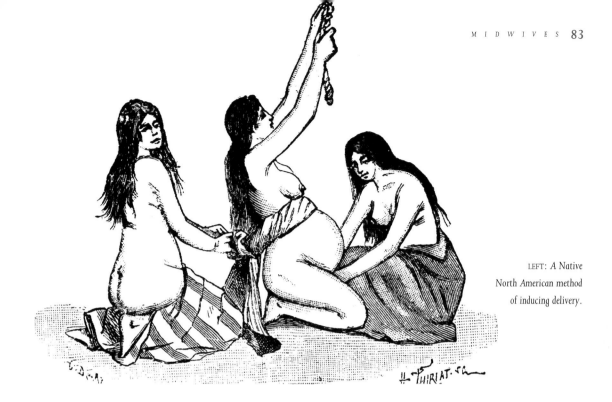

LEFT: *A Native North American method of inducing delivery.*

She will be unperturbed, unafraid in danger, able to state clearly the reasons for her measures, she will bring reassurance to her patients, and be sympathetic...She must love work in order to persevere through all vicissitudes (for a woman who wishes to acquire such vast knowledge needs manly patience).[2]

Birth[3] was known as "waiting" in the thirteenth century; friends, neighbors, and women friends would sit with the woman in labor to give support and practical help, and the village wise woman would be called for her herbal remedies. She would encourage the pregnant woman and make teas to hasten labor – wallflower was a diuretic, while lady's-mantle and ergot (a fungus found on grain) increased uterine contractions, and herbal oils would soften the cervix. Henbane was a soporific, giving twilight sleep when the woman was exhausted, and nettle and shepherd's purse helped to stem hemorrhages.

2. GYNECOLOGY, VOL. 1, SORANUS. **3.** ANDERSON AND ZISSNER, OP. CIT., PP.106–9.

The midwife would know how to determine the position of the baby, listen to its heartbeat, and with her fingers measure the dilation of the cervix. She would then push down on the uterus to expel the child and the afterbirth.

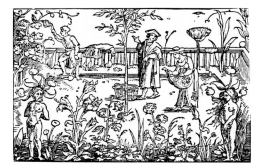

ABOVE: *Herbs were traditionally used to hasten labor and relax the woman.*

Peasant women sat up for the early stages of labor, on straw to absorb the discharges, and then transferred to the moon-shaped birthing stools for the birth itself. The birthing stool was similar to a sturdy chair, with a strong back and most of the seat cut away so that the remaining part looked like a new moon. Around the bottom was draped black cloth, and the seat was covered with cloth so that neither mother nor child would be bruised during labor. The midwife would sit in front of the chair to catch the baby, with two women at either side holding the woman down as the pains increased. Women liked these upright positions as the pull of gravity helped delivery.

Transverse and breech presentations were not rare – a breech might be delivered safely, but a transverse presentation, with the baby lying across the cervix, would be impossible. The midwife, running the risk of infection would try to turn the baby either from outside or within the uterus. Ambroise Paré, working at the Hôtel Dieu, claimed to have invented this technique, known as the "podalic version," in the sixteenth century, but it was known to Greek and Roman physicians. Lay midwives were also familiar with the technique and have been practicing it for millennia.

Infections postpartum (after childbirth) were common, especially among poor women, who started work again too soon after the birth and would frequently hemorrhage and die. An Italian peasant woman, Maria, went to the fields to carry wheat sheaves for the threshing machine a week after the birth of her sixth child. She hemhorraged and bled to death, as women had done for centuries.[4]

Noble women suffered in the same way as their impoverished sisters and died in huge numbers as a result of childbirth. As late as the seventeenth century, forty-five per cent of noble women died before the age of fifty, twenty-five per cent of them from childbirth.

The attributes listed by Soranus still hold good today, for more than anything the midwife needs patience, a calm bedside manner and knowledge

---

4. IBID., P.108.

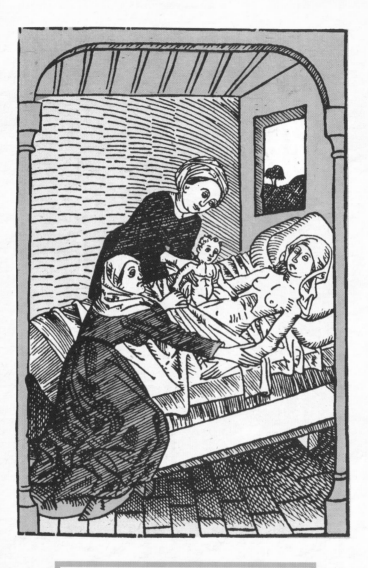

ABOVE: *A fifteenth-century German woodcut*
showing a midwife assisting at a home birth.

of the body's workings. The latter was the main stumbling block for midwives. The Church had long banned the postmortem and dissection of corpses, and in any case women were barred from medical education.

Traditional midwives are still sought out by women living in rural areas or in developing countries, where they cannot afford Western medicine or prefer not to be treated by a male practitioner. In Africa,[5] the midwives perform a type of abdominal massage during pregnancy, which corrects malpresentation of the fetus and helps to relieve backache. They prescribe "slippery medicine," which dilates the birth canal, and use herbal remedies to strengthen the mother and to shorten labor. They know how to diagnose anemia (through pallor) and can calculate when the baby is due. Generally the woman returns to her mother's house for the last few weeks of pregnancy, for the birth and confinement, especially for the first baby. Midwives also give advice on diet, activity levels, and on local taboos. Sexual intercourse for the first two trimesters is allowed, as is it believed to make the baby strong. Normal activity is generally encouraged to build up the woman for labor, and she is urged not to cry out in labor as this will prolong the birth, and to carry on as normal until the second stage of labor has been reached. If a labor is prolonged, it is believed that this is because the woman has been unfaithful to her husband, and she is pinched by the midwife to call out the names of her lovers in order to clear the blockage, for fear has long been known to prolong labor.

A traditional *partera*[6] or midwife in New Mexico, Jesusita Aragon began her training when she was just thirteen and has delivered more than 20,000 babies, including twenty-five sets of twins and two groups of triplets. She describes the experience as a spiritual one, the "miracle of birth," and is filled with wonder at each one. She trained with her grandmother, who taught her herbal remedies, how to examine a patient and how each person is different. Her grandmother also showed her how to touch, and Jesusita touches as softly as possible so as not to alarm the mother.

Grandmother and granddaughter worked together until Jesusita was forty years old. She now works alongside medical doctors, who respect her skills and gentle manner. Working intuitively, she sees hers as a gift from God and prays to the saints to help her in her work. ∾

TROTULA OF SALERNO
?– 1 0 9 7

Italian women as well as men practiced medicine and surgery, like their predecessors in the Roman Empire. In Naples, between 1273 and 1410,

5. SEE SANDRA ANDERSON AND FRANTS STARGAND, *TRADITIONAL MIDWIVES*, IPELEGENG PUBLISHERS, GABARONE, BOTSWANA, 1986, P.312. 6. *MEDICINE WOMEN, CURANDERAS AND WOMEN DOCTORS*, BOBETTE PERRONE, HENRIETTA STOCKEL AND VICTORIA KRUEGER, UNIVERSITY OF OKLAHOMA PRESS, NORMAN, 1989, PP.115–19.

twenty-four women were licensed as surgeons. In Salerno, licenses to practice medicine were granted by the state, and the Church had no say in the matter, so it was more likely that women were allowed to practice medicine.

Recent studies suggest that Trotula was the wife of Johannes Platearius, probably the same Trotula who died in 1097, a member of the noble di Ruggiero family. She taught, treated diseases, and wrote at the University of Salerno in the eleventh century. She must have been held in great repute, for when she died her casket was attended by a procession of mourners two miles long. Her writings show that she was familiar with the medical works of Galen, Soranus, Cleopatra, Hippocrates, and Theodorus. The most important work credited to her is *Passionibus Mulerium Curandorum* (Concerning the Diseases of Women), also referred to as *Trotula Major*. The first page reads:

The original book of Trotula on curing the sickness of women before, during, and after parturition never before published in which is set forth the accidents, diseases, and passions of the female sex; the care of infants and children from birth; the choice of a nurse and other matters related to this.[7]

In her introduction Trotula discusses her belief that the female body is colder than the male and that a woman is more likely to fall sick, especially in her organs of reproduction. She argues that women, due to their natural modesty, do not discuss their gynecological problems with male doctors, but with her, a female physician, they unburden themselves.

Like Hildegard, Trotula refers to menstruation as "flowers" and says, "as trees do not produce fruit without flowers so women without menses are deprived of the function of conception."[8] She says that some women will never conceive, because they are either too thin or too fat. And some have a womb so soft and slippery that the seed falls out. Modern research has found that at ovulation (the time when a woman is most likely to conceive) a woman's vaginal secretion becomes thicker in order to "hold" the seminal fluid, so Trotula was not far off. She also states that sometimes the seminal fluid is too liquid and prevents conception – again a truth born out by modern research.

On pregnancy, Trotula shines out in the compassion that she evinces: "When a woman is first pregnant care must be taken that nothing be named in her presence which cannot be had because if she shall ask for it and it not be given to her she has occasion for miscarrying."[9] Her book also contains a wealth of practical advice.

7. *THE DISEASES OF WOMEN: A TRANSLATION OF PASSIONIBUS MULERIUM CURANDORUM*, ELIZABETH MASON-HOHL, WARD RICHIE PRESS, HOLLYWOOD, CA., 1940, P.1.
8. IBID., P.2. **9.** IBID., P.21.

If she craves strange foods, like potter's earth, coal or chalk, let her be given beans cooked with sugar. As the time of birth nears, let her bathe often and her abdomen be massaged with oil of violets. Give her light, easily digestible food, like oranges and pomegranates. If her ankles swell, massage them with oil of roses and vinegar. If she suffers from wind, give her mint, mastic, cardamon and carrot root.

Although skilled in obstetrics, it is clear that Trotula is not simply a midwife: "It is to be noted that there are certain physical remedies whose virtues are obscure to us, but which are advanced as done by midwives."[10] For a difficult labor she suggests bathing the woman in water combined with chickpeas, flaxseed, barley, and cooked mallow, and rubbing her abdomen with oil of roses or oil of violets. "Do not let those present look the woman in the face as women in labor are apt to be bashful."[11]

After childbirth she describes the pain in the uterus as being like "a wild beast of the forest" wandering from side to side. For women who have ruptured after childbirth, she suggests the roots of black bryony and cinnamon ground to a powder and injected into the vulva so that the torn parts will grow together. Trotula also recognizes that heavy handling in childbirth

causes pain: "Likewise to some women harm occurs in childbirth on account of the mistakes of those attending."[12]

For those who bleed heavily after childbirth she recommends the juice of mugwort, sage, and pennyroyal; and for painful breasts from breast-feeding, potter's earth blended with vinegar as a poultice, which alleviates the pain and regulates the milk.

Trotula Major was the most widely read and plagiarized manuscript on women's disease until Louise Bourgeois's bestseller in the seventeenth century (see p.89).

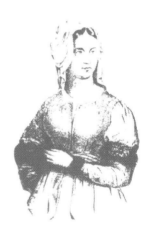

ABOVE: *Trotula of Salerno was a skilled midwife and physician.*

10. IBID., P.22. 11. IBID., P.23. 12. IBID., P.28.

LOUISE BOURGEOIS

(1563–1636)

Louise Bourgeois was midwife to Marie de' Medici, Queen of France, and was Europe's acknowledged authority on midwifery. Born outside Paris, she married Martin Boursier, a barber-surgeon, and became assistant to Ambroise Paré, head surgeon at the Hôtel de Dieu (see p.102). By her early twenties she had three children and apprenticed herself to a midwife, as well as assisting her husband. She was practicing in Paris in 1593 and was appointed midwife to the queen in 1601.

In 1609 her book, entitled *Several Observations on Sterility, Miscarriage, Fertility, Childbirth, and the Illnesses of Women and Newborn Infants*, was published. It had fifty chapters of explanations and observations. She described the symptoms of pregnancy, illustrated and explained miscarriage and premature birth. She recommended rest to stop hemhorrage, and induced labor for placenta previa (separation from the uterine wall). She explained when and how to intervene in labor and gave twelve possible presentations of the fetus.

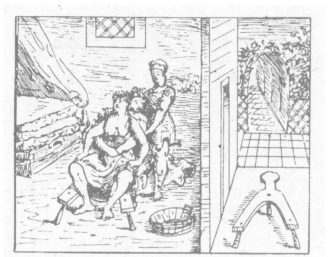

ABOVE: In the sixteenth-century a "scientific" posture for labor, using a birthing stool, was advocated in Europe.

Louise spoke out against the fashion of "male midwives," writing of their misdiagnoses, their impatience, and the damage they did to women, especially male surgeons who were brought in when labor was difficult, but she also admitted that midwives often endangered the lives of their patients by waiting too long before calling the surgeon. Midwives were afraid of being shown up by male doctors.

Like Trotula of Salerno before her, Louise called for the better education of midwives and asked that fair-minded doctors and surgeons instruct them in medicine so that they themselves could be as skillful and capable as she had been. ❧

JANE SHARP AND MRS. CELLIER

Jane Sharp published her *Midwife's Book*[13] in 1671 in the hope that "the common people of the land" might have just as safe deliveries as "the Ladies of the country," although she claimed that country women suffered less than noble women in childbirth. Both Jane Sharp and her contemporary Mrs. Cellier, who was sent to the stocks several times for her disobedience, were vociferous in their calls for better midwifery training. No one was listening, however, and the status of the midwife remained low, and she was seen by male doctors as drunken, dirty, and ignorant, if not downright dangerous.

The two women were the most famous midwives in England in the seventeenth century. Jane had been in practice in London for thirty years when she published her book. It was written in accessible language so that the ordinary midwife might follow it, but she insisted that midwives should learn anatomy. It was also written to enable women to prepare themselves for childbirth. It was a small book (just 8 x 4 in/10 x 20cm) of 418 pages. Its six parts cover anatomy, signs of pregnancy, sterility, conduct of labor, diseases of pregnancy, and postpartum diseases. It tells how to choose the nurse and how to care for the baby. Jane uses Trotula's book for descriptions of uterine diseases and problems with menstruation. The book went through several editions.

Mrs. Cellier was a more boisterous character and confronted the medical profession head-on. She was a midwife of excellent reputation, well-to-do, and educated. She realized that it would be impossible to elevate the status of the midwife unless midwives themselves were organized. She presented a bill to the king proposing that he unite midwives by a Royal Charter. He promised to do this but never did so.

She collected statistics showing that in the twenty years from 1643, 6,000 English women died in childbirth, 13,000 children were born dead, and 5,000 died during childbirth. She claimed that this was due to want "of due skill and care in those women who practice the art of midwifery."[14] In 1662 she made plans for a Royal Lying-in Hospital (possibly along the lines of the Hôtel de Dieu in Paris, a center of midwifery excellence at that time). Her hospital was to be well-staffed and clean, caring for mothers, training nurses, and providing homes for illegitimate babies. She suggested that collection boxes should be placed in churches and public places to raise funds. Midwives themselves should join her corporation, and those of the first rank might be matrons and would pay the sum of five pounds annually. Ordinary midwives would pay half that amount. She expected such funds to be

13. *THE MIDWIFE'S BOOK*, JANE SHARP, REPRINTED BY GORLAND PUBLISHING INC., NEW YORK, 1985. **14.** *A HISTORY OF WOMEN IN MEDICINE*, KATE CAMPBELL HURD-MEAD, HADDAM PRESS, HADDAM, CONN., 1938, P.398.

raised so that twelve lesser hospitals might be established in twelve of the largest parishes, each governed by a matron, where destitute women might safely deliver their babies and live protected by the corporation.

But there was not enough public interest for the scheme to get off the ground. England had to wait another two hundred years before women would themselves build their own hospitals and maternity units (see p.110). ✎

AMERICAN LAY MIDWIFERY

In the United States, which used to have one of the most repressive anti-midwife policies, the tide of public opinion is turning against high-tech, interventionist birth and, once again, the lay midwife is coming into her own.

In the early days of the colony, it was naturally the women who assisted in childbirth. They used a variety of local plants, the most common being sassafras, a blood purifier, and also tobacco and snake root for fever. Midwives traveled on horseback through miles of virgin forest to help at births. Anne Eliot was said to have been as good a doctor as any man in the colonies, and the town of Roxbury in New York State erected a monument to her memory in 1687. Mrs. Wyat, who died in Dorchester, New Brunswick, in 1705 at the age of ninety-four, was said to have assisted

at 1,100 births. A Mrs. Whitmore was said to have officiated at more than 2,000 births without ever losing a patient. Mrs. Thomas of Marlboro, Massachusetts, was said to have ridden on horseback up until her eighty-seventh year through hundreds of miles of forest, caring for mothers and their babies. Ruth Barnaby of Boston was a midwife for over forty years and died, age 101, in 1765. And Elizabeth Phillips had the following epitaph when she died in 1761:

Here lyes interred ye Body of Mrs. Elizabeth Phillips, Wife to Elizer Phillips, who was born in Westminster, in great Britain, & Commission'd by John Lord, Bishop of London, in ye Year 1719, & by ye Blessing of God, has brought into this World above 3000 Children Died May 6, 1761, Aged 76 Years.[15]

It is clear that the settlers learned much of their medicine from the Native Americans, who would have pointed out common medicinal plants – goldenseal, cone root, squaw vine, and so on – and also helped with the unfamiliar illnesses that the new immigrants encountered. Until the medical profession became organized in the late nineteenth century, lay midwives delivered the

15. IBID., P.412.

babies, especially in rural areas. But the American Medical Association has always been fervently opposed to midwives and saw their independent practice as a threat to their power base.

The lay midwife[16] movement developed from the counterculture movement in the 1960s and 1970s, and there were several starting points. Some women were averse to what they saw as "male medicine" and opted to be attended only by women during their deliveries. Other women rejected the technology of mainstream obstetrics and wanted a birth that was more "natural," without high-tech medical paraphernalia. This included the famous water births pioneered by French obstetrician Frederick Leboyer, and births in the squatting position, using gravity to aid delivery and without anesthesia or drugs. Money also played an important part – birth is very expensive and many of these women living in "alternative communities" were without the means to give birth in the way they wanted, even should it be available.

At first the birth attendants were friends and neighbors, who "dropped by" to help out and had personal experience of childbirth. Later, as certain women attended more and more births, their reputation having spread, these "midwives" began to confront the dilemma of "professionalism" versus "lay midwifery." Because of the time they were spending with the pregnant women, the midwives had to begin to charge fees to cover their expenses and, later, to reward their work.

Since many midwives were based in the countryside, isolation was a problem, so they organized themselves into loose-knit "support groups," to which they could bring problems and issues that arose in their practices. These meetings also gave the midwives an opportunity to be supervised by their "peers." Sometimes there was strong feeling, as one practitioner criticized

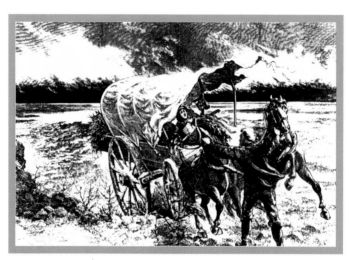

ABOVE: *Early midwives in America had to travel many miles to assist at births.*

---

16. SEE MARGARET REID, *THE AMERICAN LAY MIDWIFE*, IN CAROL SHEPHERD MCCLAIN (ED.), *WOMEN AS HEALERS*, CROSS-CULTURAL PERSPECTIVES, RUTGERS UNIVERSITY PRESS, NEW BRUNSWICK, N.J., 1989, PP.226–38.

another, but generally the women reported feeling supported and listened to by midwives whom they respected. It was an affirming process.

As their practices grew, the women had to decide how much technology they would use: fetal heart monitors, drugs for hemhorrages, blood-pressure kits, and so on. Some chose to remain true to their original ideals and used only herbal or homeopathic remedies; others felt the need for medical backup in case of emergencies. They were also confronted with the option to become licensed and to go "straight."

The aversion to midwifery felt by the medical establishment is gradually easing, and now midwives may practice legally in many states. Training programs have been set up in numerous universities, and midwives practice in hospitals throughout the country. This leaves lay midwives in a dilemma. Some have chosen the professional route and have taken exams and joined the ranks of licensed midwives working in hospitals; others have preferred to retain their "independent" status, and may be licensed or not, but choose to work outside the medical establishment. These women have much more freedom to assist at the type of births they want to promote — low-tech, woman-centered and, most importantly, home deliveries. ৵

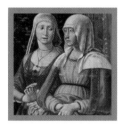

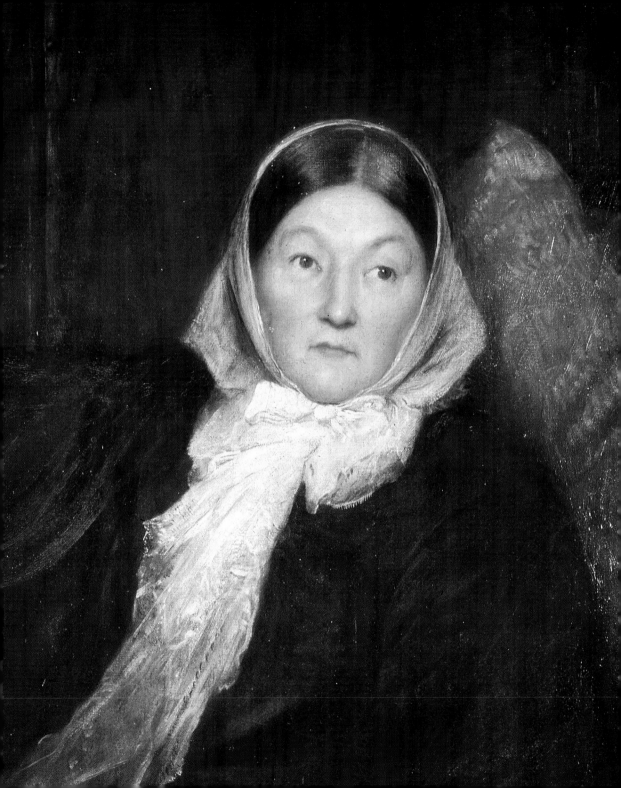

PUBLIC HEALTH: HOSPITALS

THE earliest hospitals were associated with the temples of pagan gods. Although there is little direct evidence, we can assume that women priestesses or attendants worked in these places. It is known, for example, that the priestesses of Isis (see p.14) were physicians and that the sick visited her temples in Egypt. Similarly, in Assyria and Babylon priestesses of Ishtar (see p.16) would have used a mixture of prayer, divination, surgery, and remedies for their patients. Worshipers of the goddess Hygeia (see p.97) and of Panacea came to the healing temples of Asclepius in Cos, Rome, and throughout Greece and Asia Minor.

In the Far East, hospitals and free clinics were known as early as the tenth century BCE. Women nurses were recorded during the Han dynasty in China (260 BCE – 220 CE), and one woman doctor, Ch'un Yu'Yen, is said to have treated the queen with aconite (perhaps for pain relief) and to have been midwife to the royal ladies.[1] Also in China, in the third century BCE, Buddhist monks and nuns ran shelters for the handicapped, the mentally ill, and the blind. The Empress Komyo founded the first recorded hospital in Japan in 758 CE, whereas in Sri Lanka there are records of a hospital founded as early as the fifth century BCE. Much later, King Parakrama (1164–89) built a huge hospital, where each patient was assigned either a male or female servant (nurse), who cared for them and

LEFT: Florence Nightingale by Sir William Blake Richmond (1842–1921).

---

1. SEE AGNES PAVEY, *THE STORY OF THE GROWTH OF NURSING*, FABER & FABER, LONDON, 1938, P.43. LIFE DATES OF CH'UN YU'YEN UNKNOWN.

prepared their food. We can assume that women performed many of the lowly domestic duties in these establishments and were seen as early health-care assistants or untrained nurses.

The early Christians (see pp.27–9) further developed the idea of the public hospital, and women worked alongside men to care for the sick. The first-known Christian hospital was founded by a Roman woman, Fabiola (d. 399 CE), in Ostia. Other Christian Roman women followed her example and several hospitals were opened in that city. After Constantine closed the pagan temples and healing sanctuaries, Christians provided the only public health care. Each nunnery had a duty to care for the sick in the neighborhood. The Benedictine order was especially involved in medicine, using both monks and nuns, and it was said to have founded over 2,000 hospitals during the Middle Ages. In France, the Hôtel de Dieu in Lyons was opened in 542, staffed by nuns, and the branch in Paris (opened 651) was run exclusively by Augustine nursing sisters.

During the Crusades pious noblewomen founded many hospitals along the routes taken to Jerusalem. The famous nursing order of the Knights of St. John was founded during these campaigns. Leprosy was the scourge of the Middle Ages, and by the thirteenth century the Church had founded over 19,000 leper houses, where the inmates were nursed either by monks or by nuns. The Reformation in England of 1540 closed many of these Catholic hospitals, although new Protestant nursing orders were subsequently established.

In the nineteenth century, women began to organize themselves in what became the first wave of feminism. In the United States and Europe they established free clinics and hospitals where women could be treated by women doctors. In the twentieth century the welfare state or private corporations have largely taken over these charitable institutions. ∾

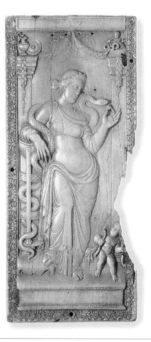

LEFT: *Hygeia carved in late Roman style on a ceremonial ivory diptych.*

THE HEALING TEMPLES OF ASCLEPIUS

In Greek mythology Asclepius, the son of Apollo, was known as the god of medicine. Apollo actually invented medicine, but Asclepius reputedly improved so much on the art and science (of medicine) that he was said to have invented it. He refined "primitive" early Greek medicine and developed pharmacology (the study of the effects of drugs on the body) and surgery.[2] Legend has it that Asclepius was once mortal, but then he became one of the gods. He is said to have entered Athens in 420 BCE with his wife, Epione, and his children, Hygeia, Panacea, Aegle, and Iaso. A temple in his honor was founded on a hillside near the Acropolis, with healing springs nearby.

Asclepius's daughters were healing goddesses. Hygeia was said "to be worth as much as the others,"[3] and she was goddess of preventative medicine and protected from disease, unlike her father, who cured illness. Hygeia was known as "the glorious" or "the light of day," and had a cult of her own, Athena Hygeia. She was invoked in epidemics, and many homes contained a shrine to her to protect the family members.

Votive offerings painted on wood or clay tablets have been found showing Hygeia and Asclepius together, and these would be presented to the temple before any healing work was undertaken. Doctors in Athens made great public sacrifices to them twice a year, both for themselves and for their patients' well-being. Asclepius's other daughter, Panacea, known as "the universal remedy," was seen as a symbol of the all-healing herbs, and there was a cult to her around Rhodes. All three are invoked in the famous Hippocratic[4] oath, which begins: "I swear by Apollo the healer, and Asclepius and Hygeia, and All-heal [Panacea]..."

The healing temples dedicated to Asclepius and Hygeia were early hospitals, usually set within a huge temple complex. People would travel hundreds of miles to consult the gods, and there were temples all over mainland Greece and on the Greek islands, one of the most famous being on the island of Cos, which has been excavated.[5] These clinics were known as Asklepeia. On Cos, the clinic is set in a sacred grove surrounded by pine and cypress trees, and there is a natural spring nearby, which has been found to be rich in iron and sulphur. The temple was probably built around 300 BCE, and the complex consisted of a temple to Asclepius, a temple to Artemis, baths, a great altar, a tholos (which was believed to be the place where mystery rites were performed), and the peristyle, which contained a two-storied building housing the infirmary, where patients stayed overnight. On the walls there were many votive tablets describing the great cures that took place within the hospital.

2. SEE EMMA EDELSTEIN AND LUDWIG EDELSTEIN, ASCLEPIUS, A COLLECTION AND INTERPRETATION OF THE TESTIMONIES, JOHNS HOPKINS UNIVERSITY PRESS, BALTIMORE, 1945, PP.140–1. 3. IBID., P.89. 4. HIPPOCRATES, THE FAMOUS GREEK PHYSICIAN, WAS BORN ON COS IN 460 BCE INTO A FAMILY OF PRIESTS OF ASCLEPIUS. 5. SEE C. KERENYI, ASKLEPIOS, THAMES & HUDSON, LONDON, 1960 FOR PLANS OF THE TEMPLE COMPLEX AND ITS CONTENTS.

Women in labor were not admitted to the compound – pregnancy not being seen as an illness – and the dying were also excluded, as being beyond help. Before the "cure" could begin, patients had to bathe and offer sacrifices to Hygeia and Asclepius (and other gods, where appropriate), then they might enter the inner sanctum of the temple or *incubatio* (incubator). There they lay down on a pallet and, watched over by temple workers and members of their family who had traveled with them, fell into a deep sleep. The lights would be extinguished at this point, and the patient would begin to dream.

In their dream the god would commonly appear to them dressed as a young man, with a thick beard and a staff with a snake entwined around it. He would be humorous, calm, and sympathetic. Sometimes he would give detailed instructions as to how the disease might be cured – herbs, massage, hydrotherapy, etc. – or, more commonly, would intervene directly and "remove" the illness. This involved a variety of techniques: he might pass his hand over a wound or tumor and remove or heal it; he might perform "operations," whereby the body was opened and the sickness

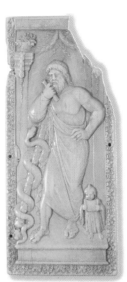

ABOVE: *Asclepius was often invoked alongside Hygeia.*

removed; or brush a cloth or his hand over the body, "dusting off" the sickness.

Sometimes not the god himself, but a snake, would appear (special snakes were kept in the inner sanctum), which would "bite" or "lick" the affected part; or, less commonly, a dog (sacred to Artemis), which would lick the diseased area. When the patient "awoke" he would usually be cured, or he would tell the temple attendants what kind of treatment he needed and would stay as long as necessary to effect the cure.

These dreams were not hypnotic trances (which are not usually recalled by the patient); rather their experiences seem to have been heavily suggested dream-states, in which the patient did indeed have an "encounter with the divine." ❧

HOSPITALS IN THE ISLAMIC WORLD

During the Holy Wars that the new Moslems fought in the sixth and seventh centuries CE, the wounded were cared for in hospitals (the Persian word *bimaristan* meant sick-place). Both men and women worked in these hospitals, with the women acting as nurses, bandaging wounds, fetching medical supplies, food, and water.

Hadrat Zaynad was a woman doctor and surgeon famous for her skill in ophthalmic surgery and the treatment of wounds. Little is known about her, except that she came from the tribe of Ud and is recorded in the poetry of Abu-al-Faraj: "I was waylaid in the maze of desire and could not reach the female physician of the tribe of Ud, Zaynad, who lives not afar."

The first Islamic hospitals[6] were built in the eighth century, when Arabic medicine really began to develop. The Islamic Empire spread from Pakistan in the east to Spain in the west, and the culture of caring for the sick taught by the Prophet traveled with the Moslem conquerors. Hospitals were of two kinds – stationary and movable. The latter followed the armies and also traveled in rural districts, offering medical treatment and surgery to isolated communities. The Islamic hospital also made a distinction between inpatient and outpatient treatment.

Moslem men were forbidden contact with women who were not from their own family, so in the large hospitals women would have been cared for by female attendants supervised by a male doctor. Wealthy Arab women also founded many hospitals. In 918 CE Lady Seidet founded a hospital in the market place of Baghdad, which had a special department for the diseases of women. The Al Mansur Hospital in Cairo (1248 CE) was the largest of all Cairo hospitals and had both male and female nurses. It was huge, with four courtyards, fountains, and musicians and storytellers to amuse its patients and to distratct those who could not sleep. It had specialist wards for different diseases, outpatients' clinics, a lecture room, an academy, an orphanage, a convalescent home, and a chapel, where fifty chaplains recited the Koran, day and night, for all to hear. When patients left the hospital they were given five pieces of gold so that they could fully recover before they began work. Hospital care was free in the Moslem Empire.[7]

In Islamic Spain (conquered 711 CE) women were much freer, and all citizens had access to education. There were fifty hospitals in Cordoba, which all had medical schools attached. Kate Hurd-Mead[8] suggests that women were trained in pharmacy and midwifery at these schools. The great Arab physician Rhazes wrote that women doctors were more sympathetic than their male colleagues, which might account for their success with patients.[9]

Further evidence of Islamic women surgeons working in Spain is given by Albucasis, writing in the twelfth century, who recommended that only women surgeons should operate for the removal of kidney stones and, if no woman surgeon was available, a male surgeon accompanied by a

6. SEE SAMI HAMARNEH, *HEALTH SCIENCES IN EARLY ISLAM*, VOL. 1, ZAHRA PUBLICATIONS, BLANCO, TEXAS, 1983, PP.97–113. **7.** PAVEY, OP. CIT., PP.127–8 AND EDWARD WITHINGTON, *MEDICAL HISTORY FROM THE EARLIEST TIMES*, SCIENTIFIC PRESS, LONDON, 1944, PP.165–7. **8.** *A HISTORY OF WOMEN IN MEDICINE*, KATE CAMPBELL HURD-MEAD, HADDAM PRESS, HADDAM, CONN., 1938, P.105. **9.** IBID., P.107.

midwife should operate. Avicenna (b. 980 CE), the great Arab physician, mentions a woman who was an ophthalmic surgeon.[10]

PHILANTHROPIC NOBLEWOMEN

Wealthy women, as well as religious orders, founded hospitals. Queen Margaret of Scotland founded a hospital at Queen's Ferry near Edinburgh in the late eleventh century. She was said to have distributed all her worldly goods for the use of the poor, to have washed the feet of beggars, and nursed the sick with her own hands. Her daughter, who became Queen Maud of England, was a famous founder of hospitals. The Hospital of St. Giles in the Fields, in London's Holborn, was established for lepers and consisted of a chapel, a hall, and two towers. The queen is said to have tended lepers there and to have visited them in their poor houses on the outskirts of the village. Queen Matilda, wife of King Stephen, founded the royal hospital of St. Katherine by the Tower of London as a permanent home for women and children, which remained under the patronage of successive English queens. Queen Eleanor of Castile, who married Edward I, gave large endowments and grants of land and manors to this hospital. She also founded the Hospital of St. John the Baptist at Gorleston in East Anglia.

Queen Isabella of Castile (1451–1504) married the King of Aragon in 1469 and is credited with introducing field hospitals and ambulances on a large scale. In the siege of Alora in 1484 she sent to the camp six large tents and their furniture, together with physicians, surgeons, medicines, and attendants, and commanded that they should charge nothing, for she would cover all the costs. The tents were called the Queen's Hospital. On the surrender of Malaga in 1487 the Spanish army was followed as it entered the city by the Queen's Hospital in 400 *ambulancias*. At the siege of Granada an eyewitness, Peter Martyr, wrote:

Four huge hospital tents, the careful provision of Queenly piety, are a sight worth seeing. They are intended not only for the wounded, but for those laboring under any disease. The physicians, apothecaries, surgeons and other attendants are as numerous, the order, diligence, and supply of all things needful as complete as in your infirmary of the Holy Spirit, or the great Milan hospital itself. Every sickness and casualty is met, and provided for, by the Royal bounty, except where nature's appointed day is at hand.[11]

10. IBID., P.172. 11. PAVEY, OP. CIT., P.140.

Queen Isabella of Castile, who introduced her
famous ambulancias, and Ferdinand of
Aragon at the surrender of
Granada in 1492.

The queen herself nursed the sick and, when her courtiers remonstrated with her that this was not proper work for a queen, she replied that the soldiers were far from their womenfolk and that she should soothe their pains.

The Queen's Hospital now comprised the nearly 400 wagons with awnings, and the wounded were nursed not by the prostitutes who were the usual camp-followers, but by "honest and competent matrons." The *ambulancias* – probably the first use of the name – were the original European field hospitals with independent transport of medical stores. It was not until four centuries later, when a Swiss man saw the wounded lying abandoned on the battlefields of Solferino, that the International Red Cross was born, following the lead of Queen Isabella and her "ambulances." ◉

HÔTEL DE DIEU

The Hôtel de Dieu was founded by the Bishop of Paris in 651, an earlier branch having been established in Lyons. It was frequently enlarged and in 1189 it was moved to its present position on the banks of the Seine near the cathedral. It is staffed by the oldest order of nursing nuns, who, once professed, renounced the world and dedicated their lives to nursing. In the thirteenth century the order included forty nuns, thirty monks, and forty novices. In the fifteenth century the Hôtel de Dieu was put under Augustinian rule.

The work was extremely hard and the nuns did everything themselves, for no servants were kept. Every day of the year a "little wash" was done, including the bed linen, which the younger sisters and novices washed in the River Seine, often having to break the ice and stand knee deep in the freezing water. The sisters' round of duties was broken only by religious offices and by two meals a day. They rose at five and went to the chapel to pray, while the *mâitresse* (mistress) or *prieure* (prioress) walked the wards. They then worked on the wards until seven in the evening, when they retired to their cells. At night, the *veilleuses* (watchers) were in charge of the wards, and the prieure made one final round.

Towards the end of the fifteenth century a terrible syphilis epidemic broke out in the hospital, carried by soldiers from Naples. Many died from the insanitary conditions in the Hôtel de Dieu. The beds held between four and six patients, lying head to toe. The doctors were men with scanty education and less sympathy for either patients or nurses. Diagnosis was taken from the pulse, the physical appearance of the patient, or by examining the urine, and the doctors' rounds would have been brief. Experimental medicine was forbidden by the Church, which upheld the teachings of Galen.

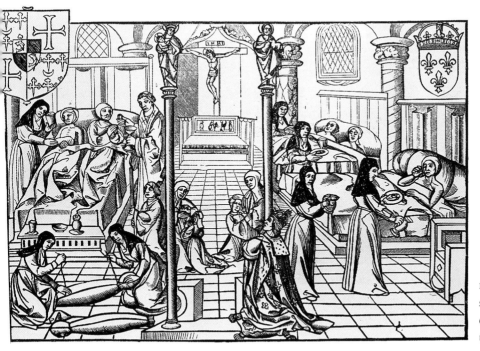

LEFT: *A facsimile of a sixteenth-century wood engraving showing a ward in the Hôtel de Dieu, Paris.*

In 1640 a new constitution increased the powers of the Mother Superior and, in 1662, paid domestic help was employed. By then the hospital also included the Hospital of St. Louis for contagious diseases, built in the thirteenth century, and the convalescent home of St. Anne, a country home for the sisters on retirement.

In the eighteenth century great power struggles raged within the hospital, and the religious exercises of the sisters were increased, which interfered with their nursing. The clergy refused to allow autopsies, the nurses backing the clergy against the physicians. The sisters resented new methods of treatment and fought with the doctors over bloodletting, the use of emetics, and diet.

But the hospital received seriously ill patients at any hour and nursed contagious diseases, surgical and obstetrical patients regardless of age, sex, or religion. By now it consisted of four storeys, twenty-five wards, and 1,219 beds, some large enough to accommodate four patients properly.

During the French Revolution, the Augustinian order was persecuted and the nursing staff became a mixture of lay and

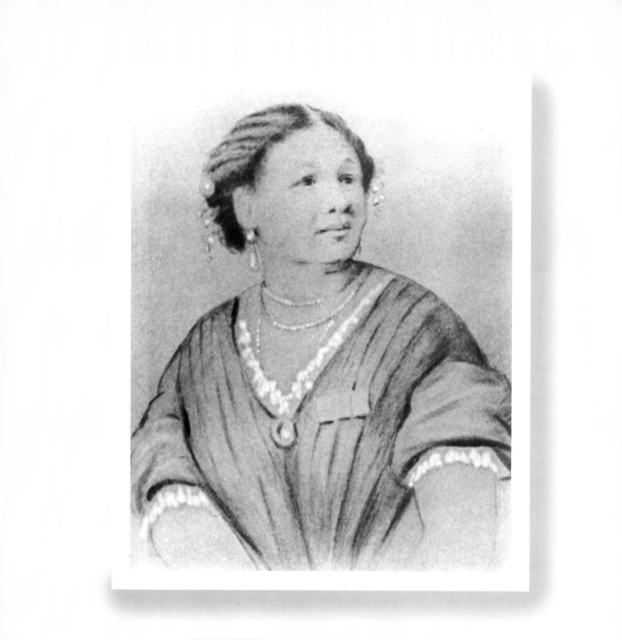

ABOVE: *Mary Seacole was a popular figure in the Crimea, where she set herself up as a sutler.*

religious women. In 1848 the hospital passed under the prefecture of the Seine, but Augustinian sisters continued to work there until 1908, completing twelve centuries of dedicated nursing. Today the hospital is laicized and is one of the hospitals of "Assistance Publique."

MARY SEACOLE

1805–81

Born in 1805 in Kingston, Jamaica, Mary Seacole[12] was a woman "doctoress" who found fame and fortune through the Crimean War. At an early age she traveled through Central and South America, was caught in several cholera epidemics – the great scourge of the times – and, through what her mother taught her, and her own observations, worked out a fairly successful treatment regime.

She came to the conclusion, long before the medical profession accepted it, that cholera was contagious, but she also understood that fear played a prominent role in its spread by lowering the body's resistance to infection. She called fear its "powerful auxiliary." She used mustard plasters to raise local heat in the body, and emetics and purges to cleanse the system. She prescribed cinnamon tea when the fever has subsided and strengthening medicines to avoid brain fever, which is sometimes a secondary symptom of

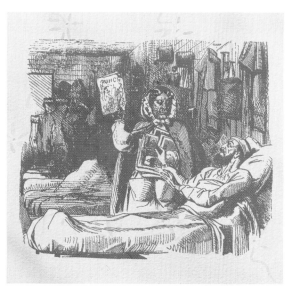

ABOVE: *Mrs. Seacole as depicted in Punch, May 30, 1857.*

cholera. Mary had a holistic approach to medicine and believed that a medicine fit for one man might well be toxic for another.

In 1853 the Crimean War started, and Mary decided to travel to England to see if she could do some "doctoring" to help the troops. Following a public outcry caused by uncensored articles about the conditions of the sick, the Secretary of State for War, Sidney Herbert, a close friend of Florence Nightingale, agreed to send women nurses to care for the troops in the Crimea. The Catholics sent the Sisters of Mercy, who were in Paris when Florence Nightingale was ordered to

12. SEE ZIGGI ALEXANDER AND AUDREY DEWJEE (EDS), *WONDERFUL ADVENTURES OF MARY SEACOLE, IN MANY LANDS*, FALLING WALL PRESS, LONDON, 1984, P.125.

join them. Thirty-nine women sailed to the Bosphorus, and Florence became the Superintendent of the Female Nursing Establishment of the General Hospital in Turkey. Each nurse was paid twelve to fourteen shillings a week and also received board and lodgings, but the quality of recruits was poor, and several had to be sent home.

Meanwhile Mary Seacole was trying in vain to obtain an interview with the War Office. As she caustically remarked, "had there been a vacancy, I should not have been chosen to fill it."

Frustrated by her failed attempt, she determined to sail by herself to the Crimea – a journey of 3,000 miles – and set herself up as a sutler, or unofficial quartermaster, to pay for the real purpose of her trip, doctoring. Sutlers existed before the army catering core was established, and they made a great deal of money selling food, and more often drink, to the troops; they ran beer-halls and gin palaces, which aggravated the already terrible discipline problems.

Situated two miles from Balaclava, Mrs. Seacole's British Hotel represented a complete contrast to the traditional sutler dive. She provided clean, wholesome food, and the officers created an atmosphere resembling a gentleman's club. Mary was "often seen riding out to the front with baskets of medicines of her own preparation, especially after an engagement with the enemy."[13]

She was the first woman to enter Sebastopol from behind English lines and to bring in fresh food. She traveled with a small retinue all over the area, her medicines on one mule and food and wine on another. The war illustrator, William Simpson, remembers her thus: "Mrs. Seacole, an elderly Mulatto woman from Jamaica, was a well-known character in the Crimea, all the soldiers and sailors knew her. She had a taste for nursing and doctoring."[14]

Her experiences were in complete contrast to those of Florence Nightingale and her nurses, who were forbidden to do all except the most basic work, mainly undoing bandages, washing wounds before inspection by the medical officer, spoon-feeding patients, and comforting the terminally ill. They rarely left the hospital.

As a mature mother-figure, Mary Seacole was loved and sought out by officers and linesmen alike, reminding them of home and safety. There were times when she refused to wait for the ceasefire or retreat, but picked her way around the mutilated bodies of the fallen, seeking out the wounded or dying, whether enemy or ally. She relieved symptoms of jaundice, diarrhea, dysentery, severe inflammation of the chest, and frostbite, among many other diseases.

The war ended suddenly in March 1856, leaving her with considerable unused supplies. She returned to England broke and was soon hauled

13. WILLIAM RUSSEL, WRITING TO THE MORNING ADVERTISER, LONDON, JULY 19, 1855. 14. THE AUTOBIOGRAPHY OF WILLIAM SIMPSON, GEOFFREY EYRE TODD (ED.), R.I. UNWIN, LONDON, 1903.

into the London Bankruptcy Court. *The Times* published several letters from well-wishers who started a fund to make good her losses. The gentlemen officers for whom she had cared repaid her with lifelong friendship and protection. She also published her account of the war, which became a bestseller. Mary Seacole spent the rest of her life in England and is buried in London. ◆

FLORENCE NIGHTINGALE

1820–1910

Perhaps best known for her pioneering work in the Crimea, Florence Nightingale had a struggle similar to Mary Seacole's to be allowed to follow her chosen vocation. Born to affluent parents, she studied nursing in England, but, frustrated by the low standard of education, went to the Protestant hospital at Kaiserwerth (see p.40) to study with the nursing sisters there. In 1853 she received an invitation to take over the running of the Governesses' Sanatorium in Harley Street, which was foundering in chaos. Her family was appalled, nursing being considered akin to domestic labor, although her father did not expressly forbid her.

Florence single-mindedly set about organizing a "proper hospital," as she had so long dreamed of doing. As with many dreams, the reality was more complicated that the vision. Pages from her notebook graphically illustrate the titanic battle

that lay before her. Her first struggle was with religious bigotry: the Committee of Ladies said that only Protestant patients were permitted. Florence replied that "unless she might take in Jews and their Rabbis" she was leaving.[15] The ladies backed down. On October 29 she reported that unless essential repairs were carried out, she would move her twelve patients into Cavendish Square and be arrested for vagrancy by the police. Again, the Committee capitulated.

Florence's success with the good ladies stemmed from the fact that she was saving them money. Her first task was to organize everything; she cut down the workforce and put it to better use; she introduced good housewifery: "For the sake of economy & wholesome bread, I have thought it desirable to bake at home, both bread, biscuits & gingerbread. We bake about 4 stone flour per week for 25 or 26 persons."[16]

Her dry humor shines through in her reports of the patients – February 20, 1854:

A Hospital is good for the seriously ill alone – otherwise it becomes a lodging-house where the nervous become more nervous, the foolish more foolish, the idle & selfish more selfish & idle... There is not a trick in the whole legerdemain of Hysteria which has not been played in this house. [17]

15. *FLORENCE NIGHTINGALE AT HARLEY STREET*, HARRY VARNEY (ED.), J.M. DENT & SONS, LONDON, 1990, P.VIII. **16.** IBID., P.4. **17.** IBID., P.15.

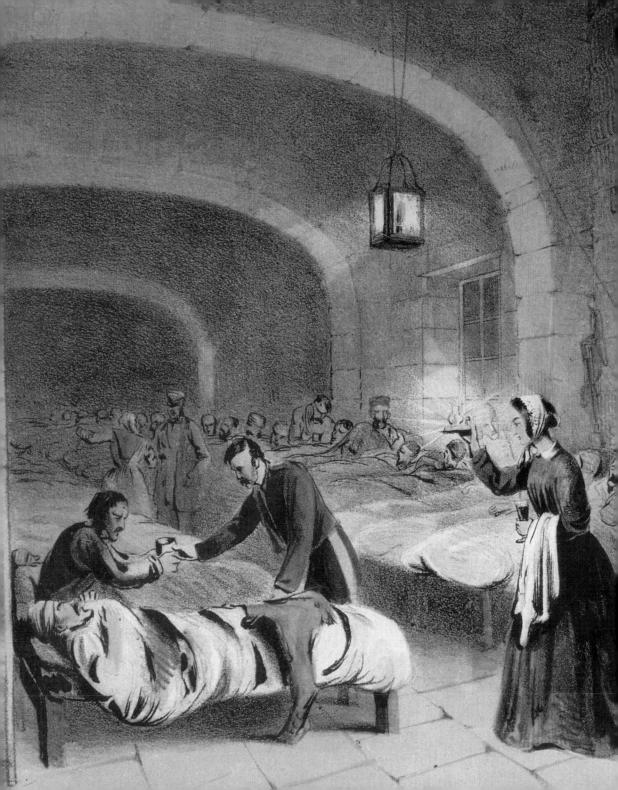

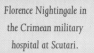
Florence Nightingale in the Crimean military hospital at Scutari.

There were only two nurses to seventeen patients, six of whom were very ill. But a constant complaint was that the patients who ended up in the hospital arrived because their families could not bear them any longer: "at least, 7/12 of the [families] of the patients have come to me & said, 'Now you know her, you see we could not keep her at home.'"[18] But Miss Nightingale had her own views on the management of the dying:

The benefits which this Institution ought to afford to the sick ... to lessen the agony of death. In no case, which we have had under our care, was the value of the Institution so evident as in that of the friendless foreigner dying ... The contest between life & death was protracted ... her fearful sufferings required constant medical treatment, by which the most dreadful kind of death was, at least at intervals, freed from pain, & even a smile, from time to time, rewarded those who were around her, to whom, when assured of their sympathy, she was able to express her thoughts and feelings.[19]

Thus the compassion and patience of the nurse were expressed in the face of real suffering. At the end of her year's contract Florence reflected on her first job. She considered that her work had been accomplished and that order had been brought out of chaos. But she had failed in her main aim, which had been the training of nurses, due to a lack of suitable applicants and of the medical cases that merited "proper" nursing.

Soon afterwards Florence was to get all the experience she could wish for, when she was sent to the Crimean front, once again to bring order out of chaos in the field hospitals. The public response to her war work was wholehearted, and a testimonial fund was started that raised £59,000 by 1860. With this Florence was able to open the Nightingale School of Nursing at St. Thomas's Hospital in London and so begin her lifelong campaign to raise standards in nursing and form a self-governing profession.

WOMEN'S HOSPITALS OF THE NINETEENTH CENTURY

Elizabeth Garrett-Anderson opened a dispensary for women and children in Seymour Place, Marylebone, London, in 1866. It was opened during a cholera epidemic, and the local people were grateful for any medical attention, even if it did come from women. This was part of a nineteenth-century movement to alleviate the terrible suffering of the urban poor. Working-class families called in the doctor only in emergencies, as his fee was high. Standards of health were appalling, and most women had ongoing uterine infections. Between sixty and

18. FLORENCE NIGHTINGALE AT HARLEY STREET, P.16. 19. IBID., P.25. 20. IBID., P.28.

ninety women came to the dispensary every afternoon, and in the five years after it opened the dispensary saw over 40,000 women.

In November, 1871, an appeal was launched in *The Times* for funds to set up a women's hospital in London, staffed by women. The funds were quickly raised and in February, 1872, two rooms above the dispensary were opened and Elizabeth Garrett-Anderson started doing surgical operations. The hospital relied on fund-raising in order to survive, and in the first two and a half years it treated over 300 patients. In 1889 the Hospital for Women moved to larger premises on the Euston Road, £21,000 ($30,000) having been raised, and the Prince of Wales laid the foundation stone. In 1917, after her death, the hospital was named the Elizabeth Garrett-Anderson Hospital.

In 1878 a dispensary for women was also opened by Edinburgh ladies, and although it charged a small fee, unlike other dispensaries, it was extremely popular among poor women, and there were 2,464 patient visits during the first year. In 1885 it moved to larger premises where there was space for five beds. In 1900 funds were raised to open the Edinburgh Hospital and Dispensary for Women and Children, where Sophia Jex-Blake practiced (see p.61). The hospital merged with a hospice started by Elsie Inglis, which became the maternity department.

In New York, Elizabeth Blackwell opened a small dispensary for poor women and children in 1853. It was a great success and the following year she was given permission to open a hospital where women might be treated by women physicians. She was joined by her sister Emily, and in 1854 by Marie Zakrzewska, a graduate from the Cleveland Medical College. The New York Infirmary for Women and Children opened in 1857, with resident female medical staff. It faced widespread opposition and constant financial worries, but provided not only care for women but also a place where female medical students might train.

In 1862 Marie Zakrzewska founded the New England Hospital for Women and Children, supported by the women's movement in Boston. The hospital specialized in obstetrics and gynecology, and practiced the aseptic techniques recommended long before by Trotula and Hildegard. Its rate of puerperal fever – fever after childbirth, caused by doctors' unwashed hands – was tiny compared to the epidemic in the Boston lying-in hospital. In those days hygienic procedures were derided by male doctors, women died in their thousands from infections. The new healing traditions were expressed when the Boston Women's Health Collective published its groundbreaking work, *Our Bodies Ourselves*, which has been a health bible to women ever since.

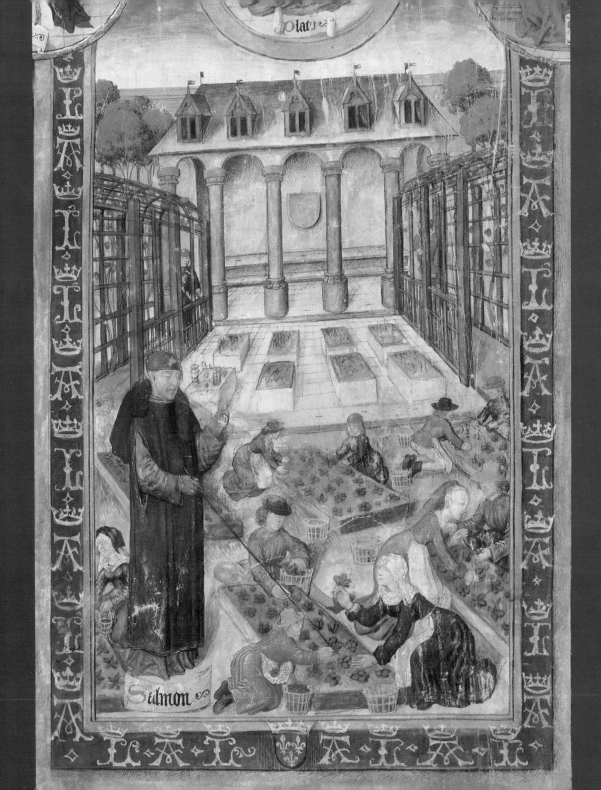

Plato

Salmon

REMEDIES

~~~~~~~~~~~~~~~~~~~~

*T*HE remedies available to women healers may have changed over the centuries, but they have generally been natural, holistic, and gentle in effect. For example, for thousands of years medicine, for queen and commoner alike, was herbal medicine. In the temples of Isis, thousands of years BCE, prescriptions have been found in medical papyri. In Neolithic tombs excavated in northern Iran, medicinal herbs have been found packed alongside the dead for their journey to the other world: mint, horsetail, nettle, all common medicinal plants.

In ancient Greece, in the temples of Asclepius, sleep therapy was used for healing. The patient took a drink, probably an opium mixture, or inhaled the smoke, and then lay down to sleep and dream a healing dream.

Ritual is always important in healing. In the healing rituals of Isis, the altar was draped in white cloth; priestesses wore special white robes; vervain, sacred to the goddess, was burnt and used to decorate the altar; special incenses were burnt – all to create a charged atmosphere that would invoke the goddess and fill the sick person with awe and wonder.

The Romans were very fond of hygiene, water, steaming baths, wet friction rubs, massages, fasts with spa water, medicinal foods, and beverages. They took on many of the healing practices of the

LEFT: *A garden of medicinal plants or herbal remedies, from a French fifteenth-century manuscript.*

Greeks, who in turn learned from the Egyptians, modifying their remedies according to their own culture.

The new Christians, fervent in their faith, practiced the kind of charismatic healing that Jesus used in the New Testament. With prayer, fasting, and especially the laying on of hands, they invoked the Holy Spirit to heal the sick. Later on, the monks and nuns cultivated medicinal herbs in their monasteries which they used in cordials and poultices. During the Dark Ages rational medicine was superseded by the use of holy relics – the toes, hair, and fingernails of various saints – along with prayer, orations, and exorcism. Their healing properties are dubious, but spontaneous healing did occur, probably due to the power of mind over matter.

In the golden age of women's healing, during the twelfth and thirteenth centuries, medicine took on a more scientific, rational basis. Herbs were used, and also

prayer, but in conjunction with hygiene, healing baths, gentle massage, and, importantly, the medicinal use of diet. Both Hildegard and Trotula were insistent in this regard, recognizing the importance of nutrition, and Hildegard was especially fond of fasting as a healing tool.

Herbal remedies continued to form the mainstay of therapeutics until the seventeenth century, when mercury and other metals were incorporated into the pharmacopeia. Herbs were imported from the Americas as blood cleansers, and the use of charismatic medicine declined.

By the time our suffragette foremothers were storming the medical establishment, chemicals had taken over at least half of the medical repertoire; sulfur drugs and chloroform were popular, although herbal remedies were widely used by the poor and, of course, were freely available to country dwellers.

As we move into the twenty-first century we see women's healing again coming

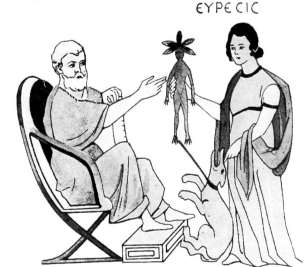

ΔΙΟCΚΟΡΙΔΗC

ΕΥΡΕCΙC

ABOVE: *The great Greek healer Dioscorides with the potent mandrake herb, thought to contain magical properties.*

to the fore, with the increasing use of touch, massage, gentle counseling, the rediscovery of herbal remedies, nutritional therapy, and the move away from powerful, toxic drugs towards holistic healing. ☙

WOMEN SHAMANS

Women have a long tradition of possession/trance work, especially in Asia, China, and India. Shamans are usually initiated by means of a dramatic possession or during a serious illness, and they may "die" and travel to other worlds where they are shown how to heal disease. They may work simply as channels for spiritual energy and cure through the laying on of hands, through traditional medicine, or through ritual.

ABOVE: *Shamans in traditional costume perform a ritual dance.*

The Korean shaman, or *mansin*,[1] cures through the energy of the powerful gods who possess her. In trances she divines the cause of the patient's illness, exorcises the sick, and removes bad luck and ill humors from her clients. Most mansin are women, and most of their clients are women. It is women who represent the household at the shaman's shrine when they suspect that the angry gods of disaffected ancestors are the cause of illness or suffering. No woman chooses the path of the shaman but is tormented by visions and dreams, mysterious illnesses, and bad luck, until she heeds their call. Once she responds, the visions and bad luck stop, and she is able to cure. In a male-dominated society, working as a shaman frees the woman from male supremacy and gives her status in the community.

One mansin tells of how her stepson fell sick. The boy's mother had died a few years previously, and the shaman felt that the dead woman was interfering with her married life. Many nights she dreamed that the dead woman was sitting on the porch with a baby in her arms. The boy fell sick with measles, had a very high fever, and was taken to the hospital and given an injection. He recovered slightly, but in the morning he took a turn for the worse, and they realized he was dying. They consulted the shaman, who said that he needed to be exorcised, because there were inauspicious influences from the mother's death. So they set up two offering trays and the exorcism rice, while the shaman sat and chanted at his bedside. The following day the boy recovered.

Women shamans are generally quite ordinary people who are "touched by the gods." Ruth-Inge

1. *WOMEN AS HEALERS, CROSS-CULTURAL PERSPECTIVES,* CAROL SHEPHERD MCCLAIN (ED.), RUTGERS UNIVERSITY PRESS, NEW BRUNSWICK, N.J., 1989.

Heinze[2] reports a case affecting a Singapore Chinese woman who became possessed by a deified general of the Three Kingdoms (220–65 CE). The general, said to be in the service of Kuan Yin (the goddess of mercy of the Taoists and the bodhisattva of Amitabha Buddha), claimed to be acting on orders from the goddess of mercy. The deity advised the family in their personal affairs, explained how the woman should meditate, and how she should call on the deity.

The woman's social position changed as a result, and her possession was seen as divine grace. Her sister-in-law, who had previously scorned her, brought her her first clients. Within a year the family's economic problems were solved, and they could buy a large house. The woman had to take a vow of celibacy and become a vegetarian. She built a large altar of red lacquer-painted wood and installed a statue of Kuan Yin surrounded by fruit and flowers and two red candles. The woman's husband became her assistant and would translate the messages that came to her in the trance.

The woman meditates until the entity arrives, and no music or drums are needed. She works every night, but clients may also drop in at any time. Successful clients often become devotees, meaning that they visit on special ritual days. Devotees come with questions about health or problems in their families. Severe psychological problems require exorcism. The woman is renowned as a successful exorcist and fights the evil spirits who possess susceptible people. She goes on "spirit hunts" and attacks demons with her sword. During some of these battles spots resembling blood appear on her clothing.

Incense is burned and is mixed with water for drinking or bathing in. Water and flowers are used for blessing, and the medium writes magical characters on charm papers in red ink.

Working with powerful energies, the shaman works on the psychological causes of disease, but generally she heals physical ailments. Clients of the shaman have frequently tried Western medicine but found that it was too impersonal and businesslike, the doctors bad communicators, and patients charged a lot of money. Most were offered either pills or operations. From the shaman the clients gets immediate personal attention and empathy; charges – if any – are low (most patients pay by donation); remedies are not frightening – massage, steam baths, herbal remedies; and the patient can remain with his or her family and is not isolated in a hospital. ༀ

CURANDERAS

The curandera[3] is the traditional Hispanic woman healer, part of a system of medical folk beliefs, rituals and practices that address the health of a

2. *TRANCE AND HEALING IN SOUTH EAST ASIA*, RUTH-INGE HEINZE, WHITE LOTUS CO., BANGKOK, 1988, P.145. 3. *MEDICINE WOMEN, CURANDERAS, AND WOMEN DOCTORS*, BOBETTE PERRONE, HENRIETTA STOCKEL AND VICTORIA KRUEGER, UNIVERSITY OF OKLAHOMA PRESS, NORMAN, 1989

traditional community. *Curanderismo* sees no difference between the physical, the psychological, and the spiritual, and in that sense it is holistic healing.

Curanderas believe that if their remedies are successful it is because it is God's will and that they have been chosen by God to heal. Some also believe that it is because evil, or the "devil, has gained a foothold in the patient's life, causing an internal imbalance between good and evil."[4] They hope that the curandera, representing the healing power of God, will be able to bring balance back into their lives.

In New Mexico the curanderas brought herbal knowledge from Spain and blended it with that of the Native Americans. The medicinal powers of

BELOW: *Curanderas, like this traditional Aztec women using herbs after childbirth, use the healing properties of plants in their holistic remedies.*

plants are less important than their essence, which can only be understood by tuning into the plant to appreciate its healing properties. Some plants reach their highest potency at night; some during rainy weather; others in the morning or during bright sunshine. The curandera knows each plant individually, understands its celestial, lunar, and solar rhythms, and knows when its healing potency peaks.

Curanderas also use prayer and ritual based on the powers of the saints of the Catholic Church, and many of them invoke the power of God to heal, or call on Mary, Jesus, or the Holy Spirit for help. They often bring their own religious articles with them into the sick room and arrange a *messita* (small table) with plaster saints, a statue of the Virgin, holy water, and so on. The family usually joins the healer in her prayers for healing.

Curanderas run a kind of general practice, but some specialize. The *yerbera* works only with plants, but does not touch the patients; *parteras* are traditional midwives; *sobadoras* heal with their hands and also use herbal remedies. Generally curanderas run in families, and tradition has it that if a child cries in the womb, it will be a healer. Curanderas enjoy a high social status and some live very well indeed from their practice.

4. IBID., P.87.

Sabinita Herrera works in New Mexico in a traditional Hispanic village. Unusually, she was trained by her father. When he was seventy-five years old and she was ten, they traveled for up to two weeks at a time in the hills, while he taught her the names of roots and herbs growing in the desert. He showed her how to cut the plants, but insisted that she always leave some behind.

Because she sees her gift as coming from God, Sabinita – unlike some curanderas – shares her knowledge of the plants with anyone who asks. She treated all her ten children with herbs, and once they had grown up she began her healing work in earnest. It comes first in her life, and if she needs to stay with a patient, she will miss out on family activities. Sabinita says that she always knew she would be a curandera. The pull towards the practice of healing is so strong that it cannot be ignored, but she did not choose her path – it was God who chose her.

Most of her remedies work so well that they have been incorporated into modern medicines: osha root for cough drops, for example, and Punchon cimmaron for asthma.

Gregorita Rodriguez is another curandera and sobadora practising in Santa Fe, New Mexico. She calls on St. Teresa of Avila to help her healing work. She works mainly with digestive problems. Gregorita was taught by her aunt and practiced on her seventeen children. She claims that "curanderas cure with their minds, with their experience, and with herbs."[5] She feels energy flowing from her hands as she begins to massage the abdomen. Sometimes she examines patients at their hospital bedside, and on one occasion took a very ill patient home with her. This patient was described as having a spleen that "jumped." Gregorita massaged the patient throughout the night and put towels soaked in cold water on her abdomen. Next morning she had recovered. Gregorita returned to the woman's doctor, angry that he had diagnosed heart trouble when all she needed corrected was her loose spleen.

Another illness common in her community, empacho, a type of constipation or intestinal blockage, responds brilliantly to Gregorita's strong massage. She locates the hard area and, with kneading, pushing, and shoving, manages to soften it and cause the symptoms to disappear. Often she prays for strength to carry on her healing work and offers up petitions for her sick patients. ❧

A NATIVE AMERICAN HEALER: SANAPIA

1 8 9 5 – 1 9 6 8

Sanapia,[6] a Comanche medicine woman, used a mixture of herbal remedies, incantation, prayer, and ritual to heal the sick. Herbs were collected in late autumn, cut, washed in running water, and

5. IBID., P.109. 6. SANAPIA, COMANCHE MEDICINE WOMAN, DAVID E. JONES, HOLT, RINEHART AND WINSTON, NEW YORK, 1968.

stored in a cellar pegged on lines. She used almost exclusively the root of the plant. Dosages followed the mystical number four – four cups, spoons, salves, and liniments, with four movements of the hands. The herbs and plants she used included juniper, mescal bean, rye grass, prickly ash, sweet sage, and peyote (a painkiller and sedative, Sanapia's most generally used medicine, which was ground to a powder and boiled in an infusion, or used in its dried state). Sanapia carried several peyote buttons with her at all times, as her minimal doctoring kit. It was the most powerful of all her medicines and the only one that she talked to and threatened: "peyote is a real good medicine. They call it...a sacrament...God gave peyote to the Indians to help them when they got sickness. I learned how to use that peyote...peyote gives me the power to make people well."[7]

Patients came to her via an intermediary, usually an older woman who "spoke for him." The patient arrived in his oldest clothes, without jewelry. The ritual payment was a piece of dark green cloth, a bag of Bull Durham tobacco, and four corn-shuck cigarette papers. The patient rolled a cigarette using the tobacco and papers, took four puffs, and handed it to Sanapia. When she took it, the "contract" was sealed. The green cloth represented an offering for the green leaves of the "swelling medicine" that was used in the treatment. The patient unburdened himself to Sanapia, often for several hours, and then she made her diagnosis. Then the patient bathed in a stream to the west of her house and changed his clothes.

The treatment began after sunrise the next day, with the patient remaining as a guest in Sanapia's house while she continued to observe him and sharpen her diagnosis. She doctored him three times a day for two days: at sunrise, midday, and sunset. If by the morning of the third day he was not cured, then she blessed him, and he left. She would suggest that he go to a white doctor, but usually recognized that he would die, although she did not say so.

Before sunrise she selected and prepared her medicine, then took it and the patient with her as she said her morning prayers. She sat on a small hill to the south of her house and faced east. With the patient beside her, she unwrapped and exposed the medicine, while they both smoked the tobacco and waited for the sun to rise. Sanapia prayed to the Earth before the sun rose and to the sun when it had risen. The Comanche see the Earth as Mother: "Mother Earth, I want you to take my words. I want you to do what I want. I'm walking over you. I live on you, and I love you because you are my land."[8]

When the sun appeared over the horizon, Sanapia asked her "eagle" to aid her in healing

7. IBID., P.23. 8. IBID., P.76.

the patient. The patient was told to pray for his recovery and to put his faith in the powers of the Earth and the sun. She then took the patient into the house where her husband or son had prepared a pecan-wood fire (pecan being a slow-burning wood). She attached her crow-feathered amulet to a beam on her front porch, and sometimes she affixed crow's feathers to the patient's wrist. The she sat on the south side of the tent, facing east, with the patient in front of her and facing west.

To begin doctoring she dropped some cedar onto the coals and "smoked" her medicine feather – waving it through the rising smoke four times. Then she held her hands in the smoke and drew it in a washing movement over her body. She then washed the patient with the smoke.

Then she picked up her chief peyote button and, holding it in her right hand, prayed to it, passing it from hand to hand, thus drawing the power into her hands. And then she passed them over the patient's body. The patient drank some of the swelling medicine, bekwinatsu (Matelea biflora) or recumbent milkweed, and was instructed to rest and to think pleasant thoughts. This treatment was repeated twice more that day.

If Sanapia felt a crisis coming on after the third treatment on the first day, she organized a peyote meeting at which the herb was taken. Three or four people were invited to pray with

her, and the local peyote leader was included. The meeting was held indoors. The participants drummed and shook their rattles, smoked the tobacco, sang, and fanned the smoke. When Sanapia began to doctor, the drumming and singing stopped. She "smoked" her medicine feather and herself, and chewed some of the swelling medicine, which she applied to the diseased area. She then gave the patient four peyote buttons which she had previously chewed. After he had taken them, he was given peyote tea to drink while Sanapia took the tea by mouth and sprayed it over his face, hands, and head. At sunrise the meeting ended.

If he still had not improved, she called her medicine eagle through the spirits of her mother and maternal uncle. The eagle arrived amid a great deal of emotion, tears, shaking, and trembling. Sanapia used its power to continue to cure the patient, using her medicine feather and the smoke. She was careful not to touch the patient, because her energy was now so strong that she might kill him. Just before sunrise, she took the patient out to say the morning prayers and blessed him. If he had not been cured there was nothing more the medicine woman could do, and she sent him on his way. Sanapia's medicine worked best on Native Americans, who have faith in the "old ways," and on those who had tried the white man's world and found it unwilling to accept them. ❧

THERAPEUTIC TOUCH

Therapeutic touch is a technique that is widely used by nurses around the world. It works not on the physical body, but on an energy field known as the subtle body or "health aura," by unblocking the channels of vital energy so that they can flow freely and in a balanced way. Therapeutic touch is not a specific cure for illness, but a technique for helping the body to heal itself.

The technique was developed by Dora Kunz at Pumpkin Hollow, a Theosophical camp in upper New York State, after she had watched a natural healer at work. She concluded that the talent some people have to assist the healing process is not a unique gift, but involves principles that anyone can learn and apply. Therapeutic touch was further developed by Dr. Dolores Krieger, whose doctoral dissertation was based on experiments using the technique.

Dora believes that we live in the midst of energy fields of various sorts: mental, emotional, and vital. She sees the emotional fields in colors. Red may mean violence that is being suppressed, strong sexual feelings, or anger. Colors are shaded according to their intensity. She also sees the vital energy fields, the flow of energy inward and outward at certain points, and the vortices of force and their energy patterns.

Traditionally there are seven major vortices, with many smaller vortices. Energy moves in and out of the vortices, which resemble spiral cones. The most important vortices are located at the top of the head, in the forehead, at the throat and the base of the skull, at the upper chest, and in the abdomen, with two less important ones at the base of the spine and in the genital region. They correspond approximately to various organs and glands in the physical body, such as the heart and the pituitary and pineal bodies.

The energy field or body, which extends in and through the dense physical body and for an inch or two beyond it, is a replica of the physical body. Any disturbance in the physical structure itself may be preceded or accompanied by disturbances in the energy body or field. When the energy pattern is broken, either at the vortices or in its general pattern, some disturbance or disease – past or present – is indicated.

The vital energy field may be dark or bright, but the brighter it is, the healthier the individual. Localized patches of dullness show a tendency to disease in these areas. The part of the vital field that is "seen" outside the physical body shows radiating lines of energy. If these lines are at right angles to the physical body, then the vitality is good, but if they droop downwards, the person is listless and lacks vital energy. Vital energy is like a sparkling web of light beams, which are in constant movement and look a bit like the lines on a television screen when the picture is not in focus. The web of energy may appear tightly or loosely woven, coarse or fine, dull or bright.

In disease it may show a wide range of disturbances – loss in the energy field, breaks in the pattern, tiny whirlpools of energy broken off from the normal stream, gaps in the web, or a jumble of lines of forcelike scar tissue.

Dora also sees the physical organs of the body, and any pathology or disturbance of function in them. She has not studied medicine and her descriptions are those of a lay person, but they are accurate, and she is usually correct in what she sees. Any discrepancies are generally because the energy web is showing changes before they manifest themselves in physical disease.

Dora Kunz worked with neurologist Shafica Karagulla on the diagnosis and treatment of epilepsy and other disorders, recorded in *Breakthrough to Creativity*.[9] She and Dolores Krieger, Professor of Nursing at New York University, then developed therapeutic touch – a term coined by Dr. Krieger – as an application of healing techniques designed especially for health professionals and the settings in which they work. Dolores Krieger has written about therapeutic touch in several books, including: *Therapeutic Touch: How to Use Your Hands to Help or Heal*.[10]

Dora has shown that the laying on of hands is not a talent given to certain people only, but is a gift that is innate in everyone. From the careful observation of the work of many well-known healers, she worked out an approach that could be used by anyone who had a genuine interest in it. A former president of the Theosophical Society in America, Dora has compiled *Spiritual Healing*,[11] a collection of articles by doctors and other health professionals examining therapeutic touch and other holistic treatments.

Since the early 1970s the technique has been refined and its effects documented by many practitioners. In 1975 the *American Journal of Nursing* published an experiment conducted by Dr. Krieger, which demonstrated a significantly greater increase in the mean hemoglobin level of a group of patients who received therapeutic touch than in those who received routine nursing care. This was the turning point for the technique, transforming it into a recognized clinical method. The test was conducted in New York City Hospital, a highly orthodox setting for such an unorthodox procedure. Registered nurses with no previous experience in this type of healing participated in the clinical trial. This supported the view that therapeutic touch is a capacity latent in all human beings. The experiment also showed that controlled methods of scientific research may be used in "unorthodox healing techniques." The process of developing therapeutic touch is far from complete, and its possibilities for development remain vast. ~

9. *BREAKTHROUGH TO CREATIVITY*, DORA KUNZ AND SHAFICA KARAGULLA, DE VORRS, 1968. **10.** *THERAPEUTIC TOUCH: HOW TO USE YOUR HANDS TO HELP OR HEAL*, DOLORES KRIEGER, PRENTICE HALL, 1979. **11.** *SPIRITUAL HEALING*, DORA KUNZ, QUEST BOOKS, WHEATON, ILL., 1995.

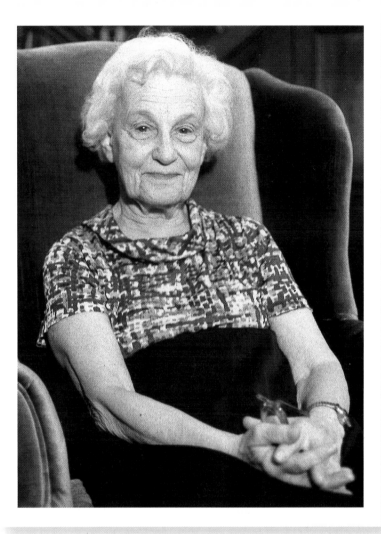

ABOVE: *Dora Kunz, who developed the technique of therapeutic touch.*

CHRONOLOGY

c. 2500 BCE Merit Ptah of Egypt is the first female physician on record

c. 1900 BCE The *Kahun Papryus*, covering diseases of women and children, is compiled in Egypt

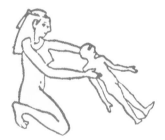

c. 1550 BCE *The Papyrus Ebers*, containing hundreds of recipes, many of them for women's diseases, is compiled in Egypt

c. 600 BCE 800 prescriptions on clay tablets are lodged in the library of Assurbanipal

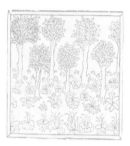

300 BCE Alms-houses are established in China under the auspices of Buddhist priests, whose work is curtailed in 845 CE with the demolition of all Buddhist temples

335 CE Pagan hospitals close when Constantine makes Christianity the state religion of the Roman Empire and deaconesses take over the healing role

390 Fabiola of Rome opens the first Christian hospital

533 The order of deaconesses is abolished by the Synod of Orleans

651 The Hôtel de Dieu, the oldest purely nursing order of nuns, is founded in Paris

707 The first Islamic hospitals are founded

758 The first hospital in Japan is founded by the Empress Komyo

1081 King Alexis founds a great hospital in Constantinople, with 10,000 beds

11TH CENTURY Trotula of Salerno writes *Passionibus Mulerium Curandorum*,

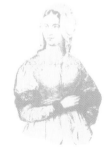

which becomes the most widely read and plagiarized manuscript on women's diseases until the seventeenth century

1141 Hildegard of Bingen writes *Liber Scivias*, followed by several works on medicine, and founds her own abbey in 1147

1184 The Beguine order is founded, inspired by the teachings of St. Francis, and establishes many hospitals throughout northern Europe.

12TH CENTURY *Regimen Sanitatis Salernitanum*, the famous code of health of Salerno, is published; 250 editions of it have since been published

1212 The order of the Poor Clares is founded; they establish a nunnery in England in 1293

1220 The faculty of medicine at the University of Paris forbids all but bachelors to practice medicine

1252 Pope Innocent IV issues a papal bull calling for the persecution of heretics

1257 Torture of heretics is officially sanctioned and remains a legal recourse of the Church until 1816

1322 Jacoba Felice is charged in Paris with illegally practicing medicine, found guilty, and excommunicated

1486 The *Malleus Maleficarum* is written and becomes the witch-hunter's bible

1487 Queen Isabella of Castile's Queen's Hospital is conveyed in 400 *ambulancias* on the surrender of Malaga. The Dissolution of the monasteries signals the end of hospital building in England for hundreds of years; Henry VIII authorizes a separate London surgeons' guild, to which women are forbidden membership

1592 The "witches of North Berwick" are hanged for their healing practices

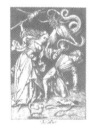

1609 Louise Bourgeois of Paris writes *Several Observations on Sterility, Miscarriage, Fertility, Childbirth, and the Illnesses of Women and Newborn Infants* and calls for the better education of midwives

1648 Margaret Jones of Charleston, Massachusetts, is tried and executed for being a "cunning woman" who performs midwifery and can foretell the future

1671 Jane Sharp, one of the two most famous midwives in England in the seventeenth century, publishes her *Midwife's Book*

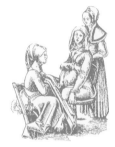

LATE 17TH CENTURY Mrs. Cellier makes plans for a Royal Lying-in Hospital, but is unable to raise sufficient funds

1737 Elizabeth Blackwell, a general physician and obstetrician, writes her *Curious Herbal*

1853 Mary Seacole of Jamaica travels to the Crimea, where she sets herself up as a sutler to pay for her doctoring activities and becomes the first woman to enter Sebastopol from behind English lines

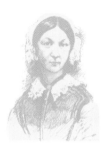

1853 Florence Nightingale takes over the running of the Governesses' Sanatorium in London's Harley Street, before traveling to the Crimea in 1854 and founding the Nightingale School of Nursing in London two years later

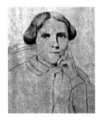

1857 Another Elizabeth Blackwell, together with her sister Emily and Marie Zakrzewska, opens the New York Infirmary for Women and Children, followed by a medical school

1862 Marie Zakrzewska founds the New England Hospital for Women and Children

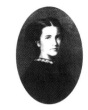

1866 Elizabeth Garrett-Anderson opens a dispensary for women and children in London, and later a women's hospital

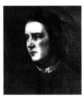

1874 A group of women, headed by Sophia Jex-Blake and Elizabeth Garrett-Anderson, opens the London School of Medicine for Women

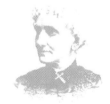

1879 Mary Baker Eddy founds the Church of Christ, Scientist, based on her faith in divine healing

1896 Maria Montessori becomes the first woman to obtain a doctorate in medicine in modern Italy, then goes on to develop her renowned Montessori method of education and development for children

1900 The Edinburgh Hospital and Dispensary for Women and Children opens

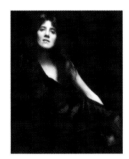

1921 Marie Stopes opens the first birth-control clinic in the British Empire

1970 The Women's Equity Action League in the United States files a complaint against every medical school in the US, leading to a sharp increase in the number of women medical students

1973 Dora Kunz and Dolores Krieger develop the technique of therapeutic touch

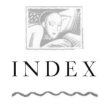

INDEX

Quest Books are published by
The Theosophical Society in America,
Wheaton, Illinois 60189–0270,
a branch of a world organization dedicated to the
promotion of the unity of humanity and the
encouragement of the study of religion, philosophy, and
science, to the end that we may better understand
ourselves and our place in the universe. The Society stands
for complete freedom of individual search and belief.
For further information about its activities,
write, call 1-800-669-1571, or consult its Web page:
http: // www.theosophical. org
The Theosophical Publishing House
is aided by the generous support of
THE KERN FOUNDATION,
a trust established by Herbert A. Kern
and dedicated to Theosophical education.